RECOGNITIONS

Literature and Medicine
MARTIN KOHN AND CAROL DONLEY, EDITORS

Recognitions

❧

Doctors & Their Stories

❧

A Collection of Original Works

in Celebration of the 10th Anniversary

of the Center for Literature, Medicine

& the Health Care Professions

❧

Edited by Carol Donley

& Martin Kohn

❧

The Kent State

University Press

KENT & LONDON

❧

To my husband, Alan, and wonderful family:
Gregory, Karen, Ted, Elizabeth, Colleen, Drew, and Gwen.
C.D.

To the M.D. (Magnificent Doctor) in my life,
my wife, Marcia R. Silver, and to our joys,
David and Samuel, Elana and Erin.
M.K.

© 2002 by The Kent State University Press, Kent, Ohio 44242
ALL RIGHTS RESERVED
Library of Congress Catalog Card Number 200102956
ISBN 0-87338-725-2
Manufactured in the United States of America

06 05 04 03 02   5 4 3 2 1

Library of Congress Cataloging-in-Publication Data
Recognitions : doctors and their stories : a collection of original works in celebration of
the 10th anniversary of the Center for Literature, Medicine and the Health Care Professions /
edited by Carol Donley and Martin Kohn
p. cm.— (Literature and medicine ; v.4)
ISBN 0-87338-725-2 (pbk. : alk. paper) ∞
1. Physicians—Anecdotes.   2. Medicine—Anecdotes.   3. Literature and medicine.
4. Physician and patient—Anecdotes.   I. Donley, Carol C.   II. Kohn, Martin.   III. Series.
R705 .R29 2002   610—dc21   2001002956
British Library Cataloging-in-Publication data are available.

As a writer I have never felt that medicine interfered with me but rather that it was my very food and drink, the very thing which made it possible for me to write. There the thing was, right in front of me. . . . [People] do not grasp that one occupation complements the other, that they are two parts of a whole, that it is not two jobs at all, that one rests the man when the other fatigues him. The only person to feel sorry for is his wife.

—The Autobiography of William Carlos Williams

৵

It is difficult
to get the news from poems
   yet men die miserably every day
for lack
of what is found there.

—William Carlos Williams,
"Asphodel, That Greeny Flower"

Contents

❧

Acknowledgments

~

As the Center for Literature, Medicine and the Health Care Professions celebrates its tenth anniversary, we look back over our history with a bemused wonder over how fruitful our collaboration is and how fortunate we are in our opportunities and friendships. In 1985, between Hiram College and Northeastern Ohio Universities College of Medicine (NEOUCOM), we began sharing visiting speakers such as Andrei Codrescu and Jonathan Miller. We also shared writing workshops led by such physician-writers as Richard Selzer and John Stone, and Hale Chatfield taught a poetry course to a combined class of medical students and Hiram undergraduates.

Ideas for new projects kept bubbling up until we decided to write a grant proposal to the National Endowment for the Humanities (NEH) for an Institute for Humanities and Medicine. NEH awarded us $120,000 in 1988–89 to bring health-care professionals and humanities scholars together at Hiram for five sessions spaced throughout the year. The success of this first Institute for Humanities and Medicine led us to ask Hiram Trustees for permission to raise funds to renovate an abandoned house on the edge of the campus to be used as a home for our activities. Dr. Alfred Mahan, Hiram graduate and retired physician, provided most of the funding for this project. We also sought formal approval from our respective Boards of Trustees; created the Center for Literature, Medicine and the Health Care Professions in 1990; and received $130,000 from NEH for a second Institute for Humanities and Medicine, which ran in 1991–92. Meanwhile, Dr. Shattuck Hartwell gave a generous gift that allowed us to hire part-time administrative help for our first "official" year as the Center.

Since then we have created several literature and medicine courses at Hiram, which in turn have contributed to the creation of a major and a minor in Biomedical Humanities. We have also continued providing summer seminars for health care professionals and humanities scholars, our initial offerings being led by Warren Reich, editor of the *Encyclopedia of Bioethics*, and Kathryn Montgomery. The last few seminars have been led by faculty teams, including two actor/educators from Great Lakes Theater Festival. We have continued sharing visiting scholars and physicians on both campuses, including Stephen

Bergman, Howard Brody, Jack Coulehan, David Hellerstein, David Hilfiker, Perri Klass, Thomas Murray, Marian Secundy, and John Stone.

This collection of original stories, essays, and memoirs by physician-writers helps us celebrate these many years of stimulating collaboration. In particular, for this anniversary year, we have received generous support from the Cleveland Foundation, the Mt. Sinai Health Care Foundation, Robinson Memorial Hospital Foundation, Elizabeth Juliano, Dr. Edward Webb, Dr. William Smith, and an anonymous donor, as well as many donors of smaller gifts who have helped us raise enough money to pay the writers' commissions and to help fund other anniversary projects. Special thanks go to Elizabeth Juliano, who chaired a committee of people to help raise funds. In addition, NEOUCOM and Hiram College both have supported these projects. The Center for Biomedical Ethics of Case Western Reserve University School of Medicine helped us bring our speakers to Cleveland, and the Bioethics Department at the Cleveland Clinic Foundation helped us use the Foundation House for an afternoon reception.

For editorial and typing help we want to thank three Hiram undergraduates who have worked hard preparing the manuscript: Bridgette Roth, Khristen Chapin, and especially Liz Wambsgans. All three have given much time and effort. For help with contributors' information and reprint permissions we thank Lisa Ann Tekancic.

Finally we are grateful for our families' support, patience, and senses of humor.

Preface

ᴏ

FOR THIS COLLECTION, we have commissioned original works of physician-writers who have come to recognize the struggle—sometimes tragic, sometimes triumphant, sometimes seemingly trivial—that is part of the calling to heal. This struggle has been portrayed, we believe, too often in cynical terms, focusing on what has gone wrong, on unethical behavior, on failures in the health-care profession. Therefore, we told our contributors that we would prefer a work that in some way describes a rewarding experience in a physician's life. The narrative no doubt would examine problems or crises of some sort, but what we hoped for was a resolution that was satisfying to the physician, that might cause him or her to feel good-in-the-bones about what happened or to feel grateful for the experience. Although we would like the narratives to draw readers toward the positive values of medical practice, we were certainly not asking our physicians to be falsely idealistic or pollyannish about it.

Our first two essayists, Robert Coles and John Stone, recognize the impact William Carlos Williams has had on their lives as physician-writers. We open our book with these two works, "The Help of Doctor Williams" and "The Same River Twice," out of deep respect for William Carlos Williams and his contributions to twentieth-century literature. Epigraphs from Williams's poetry and prose mark the changes and transitions in this collection. Following the essays on Williams is Rafael Campo's "Healing and Poetry," an examination of the connection between poetic expression and healing and of how the author incorporates the power of words in his practice.

The stories and essays in the next group of works employ grand perspectives. Clashes between forces of creation and destruction pervade F. Gonzalez-Crussi's story "Birth Pangs." Archetypal Antigone-like conflicts between genders and generations inspire Susan Mates's story "Mercy Shall Follow." Institutional economic survival issues drive David Hellerstein's essay, and another contemporary issue, balancing of primary care with specialization, is depicted in Perri Klass's work. In "Dennis Bruce," David Hilfiker focuses on issues of race and class of homeless men dying of AIDS in Washington, D.C., while Larry Schneiderman in "Have a Beautiful Day Hot Air Balloons" observes cultural displacement of a Holocaust survivor and his caretaker, a Vietnamese boat person, both of whom had been trained as physicians. In "Max and the Golden Mean," a tender and sympathetic portrayal, Jack Coulehan addresses the place of a physician's ideals and virtues when they don't match the reality of his everyday practice. In a darker mood, in "Tara Sunshine," Fitzhugh Mullan tells a story of a conventional physician encountering the misguided beliefs of a sick child's "new age" parents. This story bridges the works grappling with large issues and those focusing on close-up encounters with patients, colleagues, mentors, and students.

These intimate stories and essays reveal lessons learned in the complex practice of medicine. Elissa Ely, a psychiatrist and National Public Radio commentator, tells in the story, "Mr. Tron's Farewell," of an unexpected gift from a troubled patient. In Samuel Shem's story, "The Affliction of Flight," a physician cares for his colleague of many years, who is dying. A house call to a dying patient is the scene for Maureen Rappaport's short story "Ballad of the Bird Lady." Relationships with students, colleagues, and mentors are the focus of the remaining works in this group. The theme of John Lantos's "The Fascination of What is Difficult" is a battle between a philosopher and a pediatrician about the proper way to teach medical ethics. Bill Pomidor, a NEOUCOM graduate, in "Into the Light," tells the story of a young resident's growing admiration for the once-dreaded chief resident as they cope with end-of-life issues in a neonatal intensive care unit (NICU). Martin Arrowsmith makes a resurrected appearance in Abigail Zuger's "Doctor A. Makes Rounds." A bemused and discouraged senior attending physician, Dr. A. finds hope and surprising competence in what first seemed to be a hopeless collection of medical students and residents. Closing *Recognitions* is a transcendent parable, or as Richard Selzer says, a fragment of a parable, in which a dying patient lays hands on the physician in order to ease his suffering.

What you will find in these pages are works that reinforce our belief that physicians stand at a unique vantage point as observers of the human condition. We offer this collection in recognition of those who are both physician and writer, and in celebration of our Center that connects literature, medicine, and the health care professions.

Essays on Medicine & Poetry
in Recognition of
William Carlos Williams

The cured man, I want to say, is no different from any other. It is trivial business unless you add the zest, whatever that is, to the picture. That's how I came to find writing such a necessity, to relieve me from such dilemma. I found by practice, by trial and error, that to treat a man as something to which surgery, drugs and hoodoo applied was an indifferent manner; to treat him as material for a work of art made him somehow come alive to me.

—THE AUTOBIOGRAPHY OF WILLIAM CARLOS WILLIAMS

❧

I wanted to write a poem
that you would understand.
For what good is it to me if you
can't understand it?
But you got to try hard . . .
—"JANUARY MORNING"

The Help of Doctor Williams

ROBERT COLES

ALL DURING MY last two years of college my head was being filled with the scientific theories and paradigms offered in the standard pre-medical courses. I sat for hours memorizing lists of organic chemistry formulations, substances, equations, with no great fascination, even interest, I have to admit. I was, at the time, taking English literature courses, which engaged with my mind, my heart, both—and especially important to me, I was working on a long essay meant to tell of the poetry, the prose writing, the life of William Carlos Williams, who I knew to be a New Jersey physician. The professor closest to me, Perry Miller, had urged me to pursue Dr. Williams's lyrical writing, and so doing, I concentrated at considerable length on the first two books of *Paterson*—an account, rendered in verse, of an industrial city's history, its settlement, and growth—which had just been published. In Paterson the city, I gradually realized through Williams's erudition and skill, America's social and economic destiny began to unfold, serving as a prelude to so much more that took place elsewhere across our giant land: immigration, energetic accommodation to the possible, the persuasive, and not least, earnest accumulation—the rise of humble and ordinary people to positions of influence, even power.

When my thesis was finished, I was ready to put it aside, move on to other matters, but Professor Miller had another plan for that academic effort of mine; and I can still recall, word for word, the exchange we had in his university library office: "Why don't you send your thesis to Dr. Williams?" I demurred: "I can't do that," to which my teacher replied by avoiding mention of the fearful pride he'd spotted, and instead, pressing the economic side of things: "You don't have the money for the postage required!" A wry smile on his face prompted a grim-looking perplexity, if not annoyance, on mine. I answered: "I could mail it, but I don't feel I should bother him." Miller now shifted the subject and asked me to think about the person I had been trying to describe biographically and in a critical way: "He hasn't always been appreciated by some of his fellow poets or by English professors who assign books for their students to read, so he might be glad to know that you and I have spent a lot of time trying to figure him out." I wasn't convinced by that take on Williams, and my impassive face must have registered a sullen reluctance to oblige, proceed. My favorite college teacher now seemed insistent, peremptory, and my unwillingness to respond with enthusiasm struck me as inviolable. I could feel my feet digging a hole in his office, and in retrospect I realized that he gathered as much—hence the wonderfully tactful and gracious manner of his comment: "Look, it's your thesis and I never would want to ask you to send it to Dr. Williams if I thought you had no wish to do so." A pause, and then this remark, delivered as a casual afterthought: "I thought it might interest our New Jersey physician friend and poet, that a pre-med student here has learned about his medicine from him. He's used to people reading his poems, but he's taught you something else—what it means to be a doctor."

Yes, Williams's stories and essays had, indeed, figured in my writing attempt to encompass his work, but I was taken aback by the suggestion that the medical side of things might matter much to a poet I'd attended closely. Even then, actually, Dr. Williams was beginning to give me some badly needed perspective through the intervention of my college professor, prompted by a series of short stories, and by poems that were so intensely personal. I was, then, in a troubling bind, Professor Miller well knew. I had become interested in medicine because I was studying the poetry and prose of an American writer who also happened to be a physician. I had started taking pre-medical courses, only to flounder in them, find them mercilessly demanding: fiercely competitive students at one another's throats, or so it seemed to me all too often. I had no mind for such courses, I had decided, yet they were the keys to a medical kingdom I had begun to find interesting, summoning. Professor Miller had become privy to that conflict, turmoil, and I was lucky, for sure, that he had taken an interest in what I was experiencing, and had been willing to speak with me about what he noticed I felt, found so difficult.

I can still hear Perry Miller's words. They come to me, often come out of my mouth, as I talk with my own pre-med course students, who want to be doctors, but who wonder whether they have the strength to survive courses different than the literature and history ones they enjoy so much: "Medicine has its own challenges, no question," Perry Miller told me, "but I am not sure achievement in that profession can be forecast by performance in the pre-med studies you've been taking"—a modest, carefully worded, and tentative comment, I noticed, even as sometimes I was ready to throw in the towel, call my prospects poor with regard to admission to medical school or completion of it.

I did mail my thesis to Dr. Williams, and very soon after doing so I received a reply written on a prescription, no less! I can still see that small piece of paper: "William C. Williams, M.D." appeared on top, and under the name, "9 Ridge

Road, Rutherford, New Jersey." There were no zip codes back then or area codes for his phone. He had written in his usual scrawl a brief but appreciative and inviting response—my effort was "not bad," and if I were "ever in the neighborhood," I should "come by"; he'd be "glad to say hello."

There the matter would have ended, had Professor Miller not been so persistent: "Go see him. He'll say hello and you'll say hello, and it'll be a time you will remember years and years later." True, indeed, I now can attest, but by no means was it easy for me to follow through on my teacher's advice, so strongly stated. I did go to New York City, to visit friends, and got the courage to call the number listed on the prescription paper, which had become the vehicle of a note sent me. Now, decades later, I can hear Mrs. Williams ("Flossie" her husband called her) speaking: "The doctor is not in, but I'm sure he'd like to see you." We talked about possible times, and she told me which bus to catch, and when. I got to that old frame house on Ridge Road in Rutherford, and was treated with courtesy and kindness by Mrs. Williams—cookies and milk, but also a warning: "Bill is very busy, because two of his patients are very sick, but I know he'll want to meet you."

In he came, a few moments later, his black doctor's bag in hand. He had calls to make; he had to go see a patient soon. Would I like to come along? You bet! As we drove towards Paterson, he told me about the boy he was going to see, who had scarlet fever, and about his mother, who had "a bad heart." She'd had rheumatic fever and wasn't doing well. Her husband, and the boy's dad, also was in trouble. He had high blood pressure—"hard to bring it down," I was told—and had been injured at work, which was causing him "lots of back pain." It all seemed bleak, confusing. I was hearing medical snippets, interrupted by sociological digressions—"the doc," as everyone called him, was telling me about who lived where, and with what difficulties. I'd read poems about these folks, this city, but here it all was: a physician hurrying to his patients, finding time to think of them, tell of them, as a college student sitting beside him listened, not knowing what to ask, never mind what to make of all he had seen, heard described, and explained.

When we got to the tenement building, I was quickly introduced, and then the doc immediately got to work. He asked questions, looked carefully at the person with whom he was talking, and soon was listening to hearts, lungs, examining throats, eyes, ears. I saw him in action, his stethoscope dangling from his neck. I saw him use his neurological hammer, take out his blood pressure cuff, his thermometer. I wasn't completely aware of what was going on—I only had the sense that these people were poor, were ailing, were very much pleased and excited to have the doc in their midst. They wanted to feed him (he said thanks, but he needed to keep moving, and so, no thanks), though he did accept some cake that had been made for him and Flossie. ("They put their heart into that cooking they do," he later explained to me.) "Bless you for coming," the mother said, even as she promised to keep giving her son "cool baths" and occasional aspirin to keep the fever down. She herself was short of breath but was trying earnestly to "keep going." Her husband had severe headaches and walked with evident difficulty. I still remember his wife's description of him: "He's a young man who's becoming older and older"—to which the doc replied: "There's hope; we've got to help him get better, keep his spirits up." "You're right, you're right," the mother and wife answered, a guarded smile now crossing her hitherto melancholy, anxious face.

After we'd left, now in the car, the doc reached for a clipboard he kept on the rear seat. He was writing medical observations, I assumed, but he was also writing down what he'd heard. I began to understand words spoken during that house visit. "So often, people know what's gone wrong in their lives," I was told—and then a terse insistence: "The doctor's job is to learn from his patients." Next came a brief amplification: "If you let your patients become your teachers, you've gone half way at least. I worry when I'm paying so much attention to what I think I have to say, that I don't sit back and let myself get educated!"

I was hardly one to disagree with such declared sentiment, but I scarcely knew what to make of what I'd witnessed, even as I'd begun to wonder what the doc meant for me to comprehend as he spoke of his concerns, worries, with regard to those in the first building we visited—and then, with regard to those in one after another family we met in the couple of hours that day devoted to "house calls," as the doc called them. I knew I'd seen people in distress and been in their homes with a doctor who was attending them, trying to do the best he could for them. I knew that he was encouraging those parents and children, even as they regarded him with gratitude and anticipation. He kept speaking of hope, even as one father told him this, pointedly: "*You* are our hope!" He accepted that high compliment, but immediately called for a broader perspective: "I try to be of help, but please remember, our bodies do the work; they want to get better, and we've all got to lend them a hand!"

I wasn't then and there sure what he was trying to convey with those somewhat exhortative remarks; it took me a long while, going on many such house visits, hearing and seeing the doc in action again and again, to begin to fathom what he was getting at: his own work as a physician counted a lot, but he ought keep in mind (and with him, his patients) that larger story of human endurance as it mightily affirms itself, often against great odds. In that regard, I hope never to forget this reflective remark spoken by the doc toward the end of his life:

We're here as doctors to marvel at human life as well as assist it, by ministering to it with our medicines, the best we can. We're not here to boast or swagger— a temptation, I fear, for many of us! It's an honor and a privilege to be able to lend a hand to people in pain, people worrying about what comes next in their illnesses; but it's also an honor and a privilege to be handed along by them, to be taught by them about what you've learned! I keep reminding myself that I'm a helper—that I try to figure out what's not working in them, and what might help them, so they'll be in better shape. When they tell me I've done this or that, I tell them back: okay, I added my two cents, but don't you ever forget that you're the one who made it all come out fine. Sure, sure, they keep wanting me to have all the credit, but part of my job is to bow before them (and luck, and circumstances that turned out well, in their favor, in our favor) and to be thankful that I've had the chance to be with them when things got rough for them.

A well-known poet, story-teller, essayist was choosing his words carefully, was leaning over backwards to let a then-medical student know what his attitude as a physician was towards his daily work: a respect for his patients and, also, a respect for life's great mysteries, for its powerful unfolding energy as well as its mishaps and its occasional, tragic foreshortening. That image of handing others along, of being handed along by them, mattered a lot to Dr. Williams; it wasn't a mere expression, a trick of language, but a way of regarding himself, his doctoring life, and others whom he knew as patients, true, but no less, as kindred spirits, souls, eminently worth his admiration, his solicitations, his mannerly attention, as well as healing presence. In a sense, then, he was self-effacing as well as a "big help," a phrase sent him by way of his patients as they tried to characterize the nature of his medical assistance, extended their way so conscientiously. A man who could be wonderful with words, who could soar to lyrical originality and expressiveness, was in fact calling upon patients and their fellow citizens. "Every day my patients surprise me just as life does," Dr. Williams once declared—yet another expression of wonder and implied humility. Then a further avowal: "I hope I'm up to the challenge of their illness, but I hope I'm up to being the lucky witness to their often tough lives, and the recipient of their stories, which they keep showing me, to the point that when they get better, I feel I'm a hard-working student who's also getting a little better—someone who's had a good day at the races, in his life! In my work, 'success' means someone is doing well, feeling stronger."

Later that day, Dr. Williams moved to educational subjects, which I'd brought to his attention from time to time—the hurdles of pre-medical courses and, no less, the hard demands of a medical curriculum (especially on someone like himself, who hadn't excelled in the laboratory sciences, but liked talking with people, learning from them about themselves). Speaking of the challenges and rewards of a career in medicine Williams said:

> It's a miracle I got into medical school, and another miracle that I got out with my eyes still working and my head and heart also working! When I meet college students headed for medicine, or medical students well on their way there (soon to become card-carrying doctors) I salute them, loud and clear. I tell them they've chosen a hard road, but hey, it's a road that has a great destination, with many moments to savor, to hold dear as a gift: life faced head-on, life and all its possibilities and problems! There's the big help we can be to our patients, and the big help they can be to us!

Speaking of "big help," I can only look back on those years spending time with William Carlos Williams the poet, and with doctor Williams, the "New Jersey doc," he'd occasionally call himself, as a great good time, indeed, for me. A man of literary erudition and excellence was also a hard-working "doc" who went to see his patients in their rather modest, if not humble, homes, as well as in his home, which had his office "right smack in it," as he once put it, "so that I walk next door, and there it is, life to be encountered." We could hardly do better, I sometimes think, than follow that doc's advice, walk in his medical footsteps, let his way of seeing medical practice become ours: helping our patients, to be sure, but also acknowledging for ourselves the degrees to which they help us. "I need your help, Doc Williams," I once heard a mother tell him as she worried out loud about her daughter's hurts and worries. "Yes, I'll try to be of help," he promptly replied, but then came this answer, this plea: "The only thing is, we've got to help each other—you telling me what's gone wrong, me trying to figure it out, so we can fix things up, together." Those words, that last word most tellingly, offer us who aspire to be good doctors, now and in the future, their very own kind of help, that of Dr. William Carlos Williams: the moral center of medical practice, its day-to-day values, actively lived out—its constantly redemptive give-and-take, its essential mutuality, frankly and poignantly rendered.

The Same River Twice:
My Education in William Carlos Williams

John Stone

EACH MORNING, in Atlanta, before I rise by elevator to my office and the day's work, I see before me, covering one whole wall of my building, in all its massive splendor, what I think of as my heritage, *our* heritage, in medicine. That heritage takes the shape of a huge mosaic crafted several years ago by Siro Tonelli, an artisan from Florence, Italy. His handiwork, comprised of two and one-half *million* bits of colored glass, depicts 33 panels on the history of health care and the history of medicine. I consider it the eighth wonder of the world, this pointillist work of art.

Some of my favorite figures from the mosaic include the following:

René Théophile Hyacinthe Laënnec, inventor of the stethoscope (1819).
Elizabeth Blackwell, the first woman admitted to a U.S. medical school (1847).
John Hunter (1728–1793), who put the practice of surgery on firmer scientific ground.
Charles Drew, the African-American physician who perfected the science of blood transfusion during World War II.

Many of the historical figures on Tonelli's mosaic deserve their places; omission of some of my favorites was inevitable. For example, one of my esteemed physicians from the past is not on the mural. This person has a special significance for physician-writers: he might be thought of as the godfather of literature and medicine, the dean of medical poetry and storytelling. A Pulitzer Prize winner, his prodigious output changed the face of American letters, especially that of poetry. And all the work emanated from his medical office at a famous address in Rutherford, New Jersey: 9 Ridge Road. I never physically met the man who lived and wrote from that address, though I did come close, as you'll see. I've grown to know the man and to admire his work in a series of encounters during my writing life. His influence on my writing and that of countless other medical writers has been incalculable. His life and work are as important a part of our heritage as any of those figures who grace Tonelli's wonderful mosaic. I am speaking, of course, of William Carlos Williams.

The poet James Dickey wrote of Dr. Williams: "Has any other poet in American history been so *actually* useful, usable, and influential?"[1]

I think not.

In the summer of 1962, my wife and I drove from St. Louis to Rochester, New York, where I was to begin my internship. I'd been writing poetry since junior high in Mississippi; and I had vowed to return to it after I finished becoming "educated" (medically speaking). I still had five years of specialized learning to go—seven years counting military service. Before we left St. Louis, as we plotted our trip, I asked hopefully whether our route would—or might—take us anywhere near New Jersey (the map of the northeastern United States was still something of a mystery to this Mississippi boy). I should have seized the day, should have pressed our little yellow Ford Falcon toward New Jersey and hoped for an audience with the good doctor, to shake his hand and thank him for his work. He was always supportive of young writers. Only a few years before, in 1956, Dr. Williams had written the preface for Allen Ginsberg's book of poems, *Howl,* which sparked the San Francisco Beat Generation movement.

My wife and I didn't make it to New Jersey. For one thing, internship loomed large before me: soon I would be on the front-line, responsible for the care of many sick patients, an intimidating prospect in a medical student life that had up to then been mostly theoretical. Most importantly, my wife was just barely pregnant for the first time, reason enough to make for Rochester as expeditiously as possible. But that failure to call on Dr. Williams was a source of deep regret for me: within a year he was dead. I was to be reminded of that missed opportunity again and again in the years to come.

After my internship and residency, after my two years in the Public Health Service, and my fellowship on cardiology, I joined the faculty of Emory University School of Medicine. That same year, 1969, I was asked if I'd like to serve as physician to the Bread Loaf Writers' Conference in Vermont, the oldest such conference in the United States (and the one Robert Frost attended). I said "Yes," immediately, of course, and two weeks of glorious talk about writing followed shortly thereafter. At the Conference, I felt more like a general practitioner than a cardiologist, more like William Carlos Williams than Paul Dudley White. The single most frequent malady I treated was heartburn secondary to over-enthusiastic ingestion of alcohol. But I loved getting to know the faculty: John Ciardi; Maxine Kumin; Barry Hannah; John Frederick Nims; Miller Williams; William Meredith; and a fellow named William Sloane, Director of Rutgers University Press.

In 1969, the year I went to Bread Loaf for the first of three summer sessions, I'd published only a few poems, perhaps ten or so. But I had written quite a lot. I got permission to enter some of my work in the conference poetry workshops; in one, Maxine Kumin found some merit in what I'd written. She suggested to Bill Sloane that he might like to look at some of my work, which he did. His counsel was direct and practical: he told me I needed to "get three dozen poems published" in good literary magazines across the country, a feat I thought insurmountable at the time—but ultimately, the task came easier than I'd imagined. Three years later, my first book of poems, *The Smell of Matches*, was published by Rutgers University Press. Right place, right time: I was—am—a fortunate man.

On a subsequent trip to Bread Loaf, as I got to know (and respect) Bill Sloane, I had the chance to visit him at his home in rural New York. During that visit, Bill drove me over to Paterson, where we saw the Passaic River and the Great Falls, which William Carlos Williams described in winter:

> ... the rocks silent
> but the water, married to the stone,
> voluble, though frozen; the water
> even when and though frozen
> still whispers and moans—
>
> And in the brittle air
> A factory bell clangs, at dawn ... [2]

We didn't make it to Rutherford at 9 Ridge Road on that trip. But I said my respects into the thunder of the Falls.

That evening, I sat in Bill Sloane's house and began to write a poem that was subsequently included in *The Smell of Matches*. The poem was a frank admission of WCW's burgeoning importance in my life. It was written in rhyming couplets, a form WCW had abandoned years before, as he searched for his own voice:

GETTING TO SLEEP IN NEW JERSEY

> Not twenty miles from where I work
> William Williams wrote after dark,
>
> after the last baby was caught,
> knowing that what he really ought

to do was sleep. Rutherford slept,
while all the night William Williams kept

scratching at his prescription pad,
dissecting the good line from the bad.

He tested the general question whether
feet or butt or head first ever

determines as well the length of labor
of a poem. His work is over:

bones and guts and red wheelbarrows;
the loneliness and all the errors

a heart can make the other end
of a stethoscope. Outside, the wind

corners the house with a long crow.
Silently, his contagious snow

covers the banks of the Passaic River
where he walked once, full of fever,

tracking his solitary way
back to his office and the white day;

a peculiar kind of bright-eyed bird,
hungry for morning and the perfect word.[3]

Truth is, it took a while to train my ear to hear all of Dr. Williams's poetic music. This fact was brought home forcefully to me during an evening lecture given at Bread Loaf in about 1971 by the novelist John Williams (no relation to WCW). At the climactic moment of his talk, John read WCW's poem, "The Last Words of my English Grandmother." In the poem, Williams's grandmother is being taken to the hospital, by an ambulance, against her will. The poem ends this way:

On the way

we passed a long row
of elms. She looked at them
awhile out of
the ambulance window and said,

What are all those
fuzzy-looking things out there?
Trees? Well, I'm tired
of them and rolled her head away.[4]

When I first heard the poem, I must admit I found it rather flat and prosy, too conversational for my still-developing taste, with language that somehow fell short of the drama the scene described: the death of an elderly woman. My opinion soon changed. I now consider it one of his seminal poems, one that is not only moving, but also eminently useful in discussions with all kinds of students of ethical issues at the end of life.

I also like to use "Last Words of my English Grandmother" in teaching the writing of poetry. As it happens, there is a "First Version" of the poem included in WCW's Collected Poems.[5] The final version of the poem is infinitely better, primarily because of the deft surgery (especially excision!) the poet has performed. The teaching point to be made is "writing poetry is knowing what to leave out."

I also find this poem useful in discussing some of WCW's major poetic tenets:

1. In terms of form, early on he decided against the use of rhyme in his poetry. His early work sounds decidedly like Keats. The following fragment is from a letter to his younger brother, Ed, about a woman WCW had just met:

Last night I sat within a blazing hall
and drank of bliss from out a maiden's eyes.
The jeweled guests passed by . . .[6]

WCW soon found such juvenilia completely foreign to what he was trying to do poetically and burned it.

2. His work is *accessible*. Williams even announced that this was his intention:

I wanted to write a poem
that you would understand.

> For what good is it to me if you
> can't understand it?
>
> But you got to try hard [7]

3. Another fundamental assertion of WCW's: "No idea but in things."[8] His poetry never lacked for things, from red wheelbarrows to the plums in the icebox. He was interested in the *palpable*, the touchable, as one might expect from a physician. Garcia Lorca wrote, "The poet is the Professor of the five bodily senses."[9] That's what Dr. Williams was about, too—daily, in his office and in his poems. His poetry was not the heavily allusive poetry of T.S. Eliot, nor the intricately crafted verse of Ezra Pound, but the poetry of daily life, of the ethnic murmurings and clamor of his working class neighborhood.

4. WCW was interested, as William Faulkner was, in his "own little postage stamp of native soil."[10] Although one man lived in Mississippi, the other in New Jersey, their impulse to write about the world as they found it was the same. WCW's poetry came out of his daily encounters with patients—and that was also where he got his news, such as it was:

> It is difficult
> to get the news from poems
> yet men die miserably every day
> for lack
> of what is found there.[11]

5. Williams was master of what I like to call "the epiphanic moment," a moment of seemingly ordinary life that takes on revelatory significance. There is no finer example of such a moment than WCW's poem called "The Artist." The poem records a moment of humorous horseplay in which a man "in a soiled undershirt," in front of a small audience in his home, suddenly performs a balletic figure ("an *entrechat* perfectly achieved"), which triggers a cry of "Bravo!" from the audience. The man's wife comes in from the kitchen to ask, "What goes on here?" The poem concludes: "But the show was over."[12] In order to apprehend such an evanescent work of art, as the New Jersey vernacular goes, "Ya hadda been there." Moreover, as Williams teaches us in poem after poem, you not only have to be there—you also have to be paying attention, to be *expecting* epiphanies.

6. WCW's poems were often love poems, whether specifically incorporating that emotion or not. His long poem, "Asphodel, That Greeny Flower" is a good example: it concerns, in various sections, death, the atom bomb, Darwin, Homer and Helen of Troy, but it is fundamentally a love poem—W.H. Auden

thought it was "one of the most beautiful love poems in the language."[13] Or take this example from Book 5 of *Paterson* in which a simple encounter between a poet and "a woman in our town" becomes the occasion for a stunning love poem. The poet describes the woman in some detail, but realizes he doesn't really know that much about her, which leads him to "a thousand questions" he would like to ask her:

> Are you married? Have you any
> children? And, most important,
> your NAME! which
>
>> of course she may not
>
> give me—though
> I cannot conceive it
> in such a lonely and
> intelligent woman
> have you read anything that I have written?
> It is all for you.[14]

In my life, it is now 1973, a Sunday afternoon. I am in Memphis, Tennessee, having just given a reading for the state Poetry Society. Just now I am engaged in a pleasant conversation with a man I've just met, who knew and corresponded with Dr. Williams. I am intrigued, of course, having missed my chance to do that very thing some eleven years earlier. The man promises to send me copies of some of the letters, which he shortly does. The letters speak of poetry and poetry readings, a possible anthology WCW may do later; the last letter, dated October 31, 1961, accompanies a copy of WCW's book, *Many Loves*. But the content of the letters is overall of less importance to me than to the mere fact that "9 Ridge Road," sure enough, is the return address. I am amazed, too, at how dramatically the signatures change through the years, mute testimony to the series of strokes Williams suffered. There are five letters, one from each of the following years: 1951, 1952, 1954, 1957, and 1961. As my correspondent points out in his letter to me, the first two letters, written before the stroke, are signed "William." Following the stroke, his signature changes to a scrawled, shaky, and very large "Bill." But as my Memphis friend maintains—and as the letters prove—"he was mentally alive all the way."

By the miracle of Xerox, I outsmarted the Chinese philosopher: I have stepped in the same river twice. I have walked in and out of William Carlos Williams's life, as I never expected—or hoped—to do. Except in his poems.

It is summer now, 1979, in Munich. We're on a family vacation here, the country chosen in part because our two sons have been studying German in school; I also hope to rekindle those neurons of mine that once knew the language. I have been dawdling in a bookstore, when my eye lights on a small orange book with the title, *Die Worte, Die Worte, Die Worte* (*The Words, The Words, The Words*). The author is none other than WCW in bilingual translation. I leaf through it quickly to find my favorites. There's one, with its fresh German title and its guttural syllables:

NUR DAMIT DU BECHEID WEISST

Ich habe die Pflaumen
gegessen
die im Eisschrank
waren

du wolltest
sie sicher
furs Fruhstuck
aufheben

Verzeih mir
sie waren herrlich
so suss
und so kalt.[15]

On the facing page is the original, tamer sounding English version, a famous poem that began as a note to the poet's wife, Flossie:

THIS IS JUST TO SAY

I have eaten
the plums
that were in
the icebox

and which
you were probably
saving

for breakfast

Forgive me
they were delicious
so sweet
and so cold.[16]

Another, and unexpected, love poem from Dr. Williams, this one by way of Munich, and, *auf Deutsch*, evidence of the interesting international acclaim for his writing.

When people think of New Jersey poets, it is likely that they think not only of Ginsberg and Williams and Ciardi, but also of Joyce Kilmer (1886–1918), the New Jersey poet who wrote what may be the world's best-known poem in English. Written in World War I (during which Kilmer was killed), and called "Trees," it begins,

I think that I shall never see
A poem lovely as a tree.

And continues,

A tree that may in Summer wear
A nest of robins in her hair . . .

Then ends, famously,

Poems are made by fools like me,
But only God can make a tree.[17]

Listen to Williams' takeoff on Kilmer, using the rhymed couplets he'd previously banished from his own writing:

TREES

Of all the things that I could be
I had to be a lousy tree.

A tree that stands out in the street

With little dogs around my feet.

I'm nothing else but this, alas,
A comfort station in the grass.

I lift my leafy arms to pray,
Get away, little doggy, get away!

A nest of robins I must wear
And what they do gets in my hair.

Of all the things I had to be
I had to be a goddam tree. [18]

Let the poem stand as an example of an abiding sense of humor in a busy life,
medical and poetic.

1982: Northeastern Ohio Universities College of Medicine decides to inaugu-
rate a national poetry contest specifically for medical students. The faculty in
Human Values in Medicine, Dr. Martin Kohn and Dr. Delese Wear, call me to
see if I would consent to be the final judge in such a contest. I readily agree,
having been visiting professor at their school on many occasions. They ask if
I have any suggestions for the name of the poetry contest. My suggestion is
predictable: "Why not call it the William Carlos Williams Poetry Competi-
tion!" The poet's son, Dr. William Eric Williams, writes us back quickly with
his assent. His note is on a piece of paper printed with the same typeface his
father had used decades earlier; the word "Instructions" heads the typed message, as befits a pediatrician's office. Dr. Williams's enthusiastic response reads
in part, "…I'm sure Dad would be happy, not to say proud, to think that there
are 224 embryo medicos out here sufficiently interested in poetry to submit
their work to be judged. I like the tone of the whole thing."[19]

1983: This year is the centenary of William Carlos Williams's birth. *The
Journal of the American Medical Association* calls to ask if I will write a piece
on WCW.[20] The act of writing the piece causes me to rethink numerous as-
pects of Williams's work. I also get to interview Kenneth Burke for the piece.
Burke is a poet, critic, and friend of WCW, now visiting professor at Emory
University. Professor Burke regales me with excellent conversation and unique
insights into literature. He also teaches me to eat beet sandwiches with may-
onnaise, on white bread—and to sip vodka between bites. Plus, he provides

some cogent remarks about Williams and his work. The whole project is a joy.

April 20, 1993: This morning was gloriously spent. I flew to New Jersey yesterday to be Visiting Professor at the medical school here in New Brunswick. This morning, fourteen senior medical students met me at my hotel, and in separate cars we made the twenty-five-minute journey to Rutherford for a pre-arranged visit with Dr. William Eric Williams at 9 Ridge Road. WEW is the older of the Williams's two sons. He still practices pediatrics in the space that was his father's office, adjacent to the family's living quarters next door, in a kind of duplex. A large splash of yellow forsythia adds an undisciplined touch to the front view of the house on top of the hill. It is handsome tower-ing Victorian clapboard, tan with a trim of light and darker brown. At the entrance, the number "9" appears in two places, so there can be no mistaking that this is the place. Our group is directed around to the left, to the "medical" entrance. We perch on chairs in the waiting room. Then we hear William Eric's voice crackling from the inner clinic and he appears in the waiting room. He is a wiry man whose facial features and general build are clearly indebted to his father's genes. Even his voice is wiry, plain-spoken and sure of itself: the voice a parent would like to have in a pediatrician. When I talked with WEW a few weeks ago about our coming by to see him, I didn't have any idea how many students might be coming with me. He is a bit surprised at our number: "Are all these folks interested in poetry?" he asks.

Our tour begins with the waiting room, which played a considerable role in WCW's practice, we are told. WCW (in contrast to his son) worked alone: no receptionist, no nurse, no one but the doctor himself, who made a lot of house calls in those days, in addition to keeping office hours. WCW also delivered a lot of babies, some three thousand in all! Often enough, as WEW recalls, the family would hear the ambulance screaming from a long way off; WCW would receive a desperate call for assistance and rush over from the living quarters. If the waiting room was empty, the attendants would simply place the stretcher on the floor whereupon nature would take its (usually) inevitable course, with WCW "catching" the baby as the woman pushed. It was the ready-made stuff of poems, delivered by an ambulance right to the door.

We continue through the office, which is full of artistic energy. WCW, of course, was deeply moved by the art and artists of his time—Charles Demuth, Marsden Hartley, Wassily Kandinsky, Charles Sheeler. The colorful drawings and art on the walls of the examining rooms reflect the young nature of the patient population. "Gotta keep 'em smiling," says a young smiling William Eric. At the back of the office suite, there is a small room where WCW did a lot of his typing. WEW recalls that he and his brother often went to sleep to the clacking of their father's typewriter, then woke the following morning to the same sound. I feel privileged to be in the room despite WEW's warning that now "it's just a regular office." "But," I demurred, "there must be some of your father's atoms around the place." "I expect so," he replied, grinning: "He did tend to sneeze quite vigorously!"

A reproduction of Charles Demuth's painting, "I Saw the Figure 5 in Gold," hangs on the dining room wall. It originated as a response to one of WCW's short poems, "The Great Figure,"[21] about a flashing red fire truck with a big gold "5" on its side, roaring down 9th Avenue in New York. Our group stood around the dining room table while WEW pointed out just where each family member sat at mealtimes.

Then to the second floor. The ascent is dominated by a huge mural, the work of a family member—the mural is a view of New York Avenue from New York Hospital, where WEW did some of his training. The second floor is most notable for "the north room," scene of one of my favorite Williams poems, "Danse Russe." In that poem, in that room, the poet depicts himself dancing "naked, grotesquely" in front of the mirror. He is singing softly to himself, "I am lonely, lonely. / I was born to be lonely, / I am best so!" The poem ends with the perfect rhetorical question for our tour group:

> Who shall say I am not
> the happy genius of my household?[22]

Not one of us, certainly.

Finally, the attic, to which WCW retreated when he needed extra peace and quiet. Cluttered and dusty now, it is most memorable for a display of highly idiosyncratic newspaper articles and postcards that WCW chose to tack on the walls. WCW, in his work, was a kind of collage artist: in his long poem, *Paterson*, especially, he juxtaposes newspaper articles, letters, grocery lists, prose, and poetry, to excellent, if unpredictable, effect. Especially poignant on the walls is a long graph of the declining Dow Jones stock average during the Great Depression. I think of what Dr. Williams once wrote, that he never had a "money practice."[23] No doubt he experienced the pain of the Depression years in the same ways my grandfather-doctor and his family did back in Mississippi, hurting on his own postage stamp of soil.

The tour is coming to a close. In the living room, WEW is joined by his wife, Mimi. They show us the leather-bound volumes of his work that WCW gave to his wife, Flossie. The numerous photographs on the walls alone would take a month to put into perspective: one is of Ezra Pound, instantly recognizable because of the shock of unruly hair on his head. And family photo-graphs: WEW and Paul; WCW's English grandmother; WCW as an intern and as a dapper young physician in practice.

On the way out, I ask WEW to inscribe a copy of his father's *Doctor Stories*, for which he'd written a loving and well-crafted afterword. As he scribbles his name, he tells me he's written a biography of his father, a "biography from a son's point of view," he said. I congratulate him. I shake his hand. Before I leave, though, I take one last photograph of William Eric Williams, hands in his pockets, in the doorway to 9 Ridge Road. After the flash, he asks me, "Did you get the '9' in the picture?"

I did. Absolutely. After so long a time, I did.

ENDNOTES

1. James Dickey, *Babel to Byzantium* (New York: Farrar, Straus, Giroux, 1968), 191.

2. William Carlos Williams, "Paterson: The Falls," *The Collected Poems of William Carlos Williams*, vol. 2: *1939–1962* (New York: New Directions Press, 1988), 57.

3. John Stone, *The Smell of Matches* (1972; rpt., Baton Rouge: Louisiana State University Press, 1988), 32 .

4. WCW, "Last Words of my English Grandmother," *The Collected Poems of William Carlos Williams*, vol. 1: *1909–1939* (New York: New Directions Press, 1986), 464.

5. WCW, "Last Words of my English Grandmother" (first version), *Collected Poems* 1:253.

6. John Thirlwall, ed., *Selected Letters of William Carlos Williams* (New York: New Directions Press, 1984), 11.

7. WCW, from "January Morning," *Collected Poems* 1:100.

8. WCW, *Paterson*, book 1 (New York: New Directions Press, 1963), 14.

9. Federico Garcia Lorca, quoted in *Western Wind*, ed. John Frederick Nims (New York: McGraw Hill, 1992), 5.

10. William Faulkner, interview with Jean Stein vanden Heuvel, in *Lion in the Garden: interviews with William Faulkner, 1926–1962*, ed. James B. Meriwether and Michael Millgate (New York: Random House, 1968), 255.

11. WCW, "Asphodel, That Greeny Flower," *Collected Poems* 2:310.

12. WCW, "The Artist" *Collected Poems* 2:267.

13. Edward Mendelson, *Later Auden* (New York: Farrar Straus, Giroux, 1999), 453.

14. WCW, "There is a woman in our town," *Paterson*, book 5:255.

15. WCW, *Die Worte, die Worte, die Worte, Gedichte, William Carlos Williams* (poems of WCW), trans. Hans Magnus Enzensberger (Frankfurt: SuhrkampVerlag, 1962), 93.

16. WCW, "This is Just to Say," *Collected Poems* 1:372.

17. Joyce Kilmer, "Trees," *Trees and Other Poems* (New York: George H. Doran Company, 1914).

18. *William Carlos Williams: Papers by Kenneth Burke (and others)*, Charles Angoff, ed. (Rutherford, NJ: Fairleigh Dickinson University Press, 1974), 28.

19. William Eric Williams, letter to Delese Wear, ca. 1980.

20. John Stone, "A Lifetime of Careful Listening: A Centennial Retrospective on the work of

Williams Carlos Williams (1883–1963)," *Journal of the American Medical Association* 250, no. 11 (Sept. 16, 1983):1421–25.

21. WCW, "The Great Figure," *Collected Poems* 1:174.

22. WCW, "Danse Russe," *Collected Poems* 1:86.

23. WCW, "The Practice," *The Autobiography of William Carlos Williams* (New York: New Directions Press, 1967), 356.

Healing and Poetry: Representations of Illness in Contemporary American Poetry

Rafael Campo

During 1994, my second year of internal medicine residency training at the University of California, San Francisco (UCSF), two of my best writer-friends were diagnosed with breast cancer, and another died of AIDS. At each difficult stage of diagnosis and treatment, all three of them recounted to me the great sustenance they found in writing poetry, and in the poems of others who had responded to illness before them; at the same time, they remarked how in many instances they felt disconnected from their physicians, who generally seemed more interested in the disease entities they treated than in the experiences of my friends. The purpose of this essay is to familiarize you with some of the writing my friends found so useful and so powerful; I hope to convince you of the enduring therapeutic value of the ancient art of poetry, even in the arena of today's technologically advanced medical world.

I propose to accomplish these goals by covering (by no means exhaustively) the following areas: First, I will discuss the use of words as a medium for healing through the ages and across the globe. Second, I will review the practices of modern-day bibliotherapy, commonly employed as an adjunct to psychiatric care in many mental health care settings. Third, I will consider the question of the actual ways in which poetry might indeed be therapeutic. Fourth, I will teach you about prosody, the basic science of poetry, which we will use as a tool in the interpretation of specific poems. After a discussion of four major American poets—two whose work deals with two common and devastating illnesses of our time, breast cancer and AIDS, and two others who are also physicians—I will conclude with proposals for more effective methods for integrating literature into the training of medical students and residents, and into our own practice of the art of medicine, in the hopes of creating, or abetting, physicians who are more humane and empathic, perhaps, than those encountered by my friends.

Language and poetry have been important modalities for healing throughout history and in many different cultures, even after the advent of a more sophisticated understanding of human anatomy and pathophysiology; in some instances, poetry flourished as a response to the alienation and fear engendered by scientific advancement. Incantation and poetry were especially important in many Native American cultures; three examples that have been particularly well documented seem worthy of mention here. Cabeza de Vaca, a sixteenth-century Spanish explorer, provided the first detailed written record of the healing practices of indigenous people in his "Relacion," published in Spain in 1557. He himself adopted the techniques of the Capoque Indians, who we now know inhabited for approximately two-thousand years the Gulf Coast of present-day Texas; he describes, in language notable for its lyricism, how he grew to be highly esteemed among them by curing abdominal pain, puncture wounds, and even reviving the dead by blowing breath and praying over the afflicted person's body and thereby casting out the illness. The Navajo "night chant," a centuries-old poem passed down orally through countless generations, integrates the human body into the larger natural world and addresses the spiritual implications of physical illness. Calling upon the stars, the moon, the sky, the sun, the corn, and the land, all in the context of the sufferer's community, it relies for its therapeutic effect upon the belief in what scholars have termed "the magical instrumentality of the voice." The Iroquois "condolence ritual," whose ceremonial incantation was led by a medicine man or shaman, made use of similar tenets of Native American belief systems; the condolence ritual, however, dealt more specifically with grieving and depression in the wake of the loss of a loved one. In summary, these and many other Native American healing traditions employed performative language. Healing was understood in the holistic sense; that is, not just applying to the physical but also to the emotional, spiritual, and communal realms. Accounts exist of dramatic cures effected by these practices.

The ancient Greeks, whose highly evolved culture forms the foundation of our own, also believed poetry and healing to be inextricably interrelated. The crucial importance of this relationship was clearly represented in their theology. Apollo, the most revered and awesome deity in the Greek pantheon, was god of both poetry and healing; among his symbols were the lyre (the harp-like instrument whose music often accompanied the utterance of poetry) and the staff, which retains to this day its identification with medicine; his son, Aesculapius, was the god associated with physicians and was believed to have invented the art of medicine; the Muses, the seven goddesses responsible for inspiring poets, musicians, and artists in their crafts, were his daughters. The shrine of Aesculapius at the ancient site of Epiduarus, said to be among the most beautiful in all of Greece, demonstrates in its physical construction the inseparability of poetry and medicine: the *abaton*, where supplicants slept in anticipation of a cure, which would come to them in the form of a dream, was immediately adjacent to the *tholos*, or theater, where the great dramatic poems of Greek culture were performed. The catharsis, or emotional turning point in these tragedies, was often linked either to physical healing or physical affliction.

Much in the Judeo-Christian tradition also joins poetic utterance and healing. Biblical poetry, such as that in Psalms and the Song of Solomon, makes frequent reference to the physical body and contains many prayers for the healing of conditions as varied as depression and infertility. Some of these traditions continue to have expression in the current day. For example, faith healing thrives in many revivalist and fundamentalist churches across our country, and the formal teachings of Christian Scientists rely strictly upon prayer for the treatment of illness. Christ himself, who some theologians and scholars believe bears a distinct resemblance to the Greeks' Apollo, is often shown in the Bible to have healed with only words; most dramatically, he revives Lazarus with a simple, divinely fluid pronouncement. Gerard Manley Hopkins, a religious poet of the 1800s, repeatedly imagines Christ as both a poet and a healer, and Christ acts often as powerful muse not only for him, but also for many other devotional poets.

After the revolutionary development of the printing press, as medicine concomitantly evolved into a more rigorous science and scientific disciplines in general laid greater claim to the human imagination, the relationship between words and healing changed but, it is important to note, did not disappear. Books only began to be used more formally in medical contexts; in the 1700s in Europe, for example, reading was often prescribed as "moral treatment for the insane," as one physician of the time wrote. Indeed, books became such an important antidote to the increasingly alienating times of the Industrial Revolution, which with its new technologies also brought new diseases and centralized hospitals, that the renowned physician Benjamin Rush in planning his Pennsylvania Hospital of 1810 established a library so that inpatients could read on subjects prescribed by their physicians. (Rush's Pennsylvania Hospital, most will recall, is considered the precursor of the modern, centralized American hospital.)

This practice of prescribing literature to patients as a form of therapy continues today in what is called *bibliotherapy*. In a recent review of bibliotherapy that appeared in the *Canadian Journal of Psychiatry*, Katz and Watt define modern bibliotherapy as "the guided use of reading, usually as an adjunct to psychotherapy in mental health care settings, for learning about and developing insights into illness, and for stimulating catharsis, to aid in the healing process." These authors describe a number of conditions in the treatment of which bibliotherapy has proved successful, from social phobias to depression. (Least surprising of these, perhaps, is sexual dysfunction, which supports the age-old belief that poetry is especially effective in wooing and inspiring potential lovers.)

There even exists in the literature a report of a randomized controlled trial of bibliotherapy in chronic schizophrenic patients, which purports to show that chronic schizophrenics who were randomized to thrice weekly reading sessions that included poetry exhibited less behavioral problems than those who received usual care. While the author does not explain in detail the nature of the improvement in patient attitudes, the results are intriguing nonetheless, particularly in light of some of the long-standing theories regarding the therapeutic effect of psychoanalysis. Among analysts, one school of thought holds that the efficacy of psychotherapy lies in its ability to provide critical form and structure to disturbed thought processes, thereby helping to create the meaning and insight so useful to the psychiatrically ill patient.

Perhaps more relevant to general medical practice, just within the last year, another randomized controlled trial appeared in the *Journal of the American Medical Association* (JAMA). The JAMA study showed that among patients with chronic and debilitating medical conditions such as asthma and rheumatoid arthritis, those who wrote creatively about their illness reported fewer symptoms and exhibited less disability than those receiving standard treatments alone.

Such research raises the question: Why might poetry be therapeutic? Though the breadth of historical examples of the marriage between poetry and healing is interesting and perhaps even compelling, and the continued successful use of literature in psychiatric and some medical settings is suggestive, precious little of this "scientific data" we so adamantly insist upon exists to support its effectiveness.

From my own experience as both a physician and poet, I have developed a set of principles by which I believe poetry may indeed exert a powerful therapeutic force for people living with illness. While I have not yet resorted to writing poems on my patients' prescriptions instead of the names and doses of antiretrovirals for AIDS patients, say, or alpha-interferon for chronic hepatitis C patients, or any of a number of other drugs that we use because we hope they might help but that have less than completely curative effects, I do engage many of my patients in a program of relevant reading that I believe educates me as much as it does them. (And incidentally, even *really* bad poetry has no toxic side effects.)

What follows is my list, with the up-front admission that rigorously testing any of these proposed mechanisms of action would be difficult, indeed. I should note, however, that some of these are well accepted in psychiatric and behavioral medicine circles. Any experienced care provider has observed the therapeutic effect of simply *assigning a name* to a patient's disquieting symptoms and signs; imagine amplifying that effect by allowing the patient to discover and to name for him or herself what the affliction is. *Creating metaphors* in poetry is a process similar to the healing process, in that it involves an imaginative translocation from one state to another. The poem, in its rhythms and rhymes, can metaphorically *restore the sufferer's sense of control* over deranged bodily functions. At the same time, poetry places the patient in direct *communication* with others who have suffered with a disease, across centuries and across cultures. Writing poetry specifically and dramatically *establishes the patient's authority* in the setting of illness, an authority so often wrested from him or her by those of us in the medical establishment. Poetry also *empowers through the construction of identity,* as the patient after naming and then authoring his or her illness finally identifies with the illness. Perhaps most important, the poem provides a nonjudgmental space to *explore and accept* death as one possible ending to the patient's life story, an outcome we are notoriously inept at helping patients to understand. Finally, the written legacy of poetry *teaches* all those who will encounter it not only about the illness itself, from a perspective different from that found in textbooks, but also more importantly provides precious details of the human experience of illness.

Before I move to a discussion of specific poetic works that will help illustrate these points, it might be useful to review the nuts and bolts of poetry or what might be called, especially for those who saw biology as a refuge from an ill-taught English class, the "basic science" of poetry. Also known as prosody, the internal workings of poems are as accessible as the human heartbeat.

One fundamental distinction to be made on first approaching a poem is between formal and free verse. *Formal poetry* observes the rules of prosody, making use of meter, rhyme, and stanzaic structure to convey meaning; *free verse* achieves its effects at least in part by breaking those same rules. Contemporary "formalists" usually write in received forms, for example the sonnet, *terza rima,* or Sapphics, and sometimes in new forms of their own invention; in free verse, the only guidelines are the natural structures in the cadences of speech and the complexities of syntax. My own primary interest as a poet and a physician has been in formal poetry, because in the familiar forms developed over the centuries I hear most clearly articulated the innate rhythms of the physical body.

The basic structural unit in formal poetry, *the foot,* is a metrical unit comprised of groups of stressed and unstressed syllables. The most common foot is the *iamb,* an unstressed followed by a stressed syllable, much like the lub-*dub* we hear with our stethoscopes when we auscultate heart sounds. *Iambic pentameter* refers to a longer metrical structure in which each line is composed of five iambic, or unstressed-stressed, feet; a four-footed line would be iambic tetrameter, a three-footed line iambic trimeter, etc. It is easy to generate examples of iambic pentameter, the most ubiquitous line of formal verse, because much of our spontaneous speech is iambic. "Shall I compare thee to a summer's day?" is a well-known example from one of Shakespeare's sonnets; "a cup of coffee and a slice of toast," less lofty in its diction and its content, has the same metrical structure. Several variations on this standard metrical foot appear commonly in iambic poetry: the trochee is the opposite of the standard iamb, with a stressed followed by an unstressed syllable; the anapest, two unstressed followed by a stressed syllable; the dactyl, a stressed syllable followed by two unstressed syllables; the spondee, two stressed syllables in sequence (which is a rare foot in English); and the pyrrhic, two unstressed syllables in sequence. *let* me *not* to the *mar*riage of *true minds* / Ad*mit* im*ped*iments, another famous line from Shakespeare, illustrates some of these—I will leave it as an exercise for the reader to figure out which ones! Stanzas in poetry are essentially analogous to paragraphs in prose; stanzaic breaks, however, where text gives way to the open space of the page, provide opportunities for dramatic effects. Straight rhyme is fairly self-explanatory; however, in addition to the most obvious end rhymes, readers of poetry should also be alert to internal rhyming, which refers to rhymes that occur within single lines, or between lines not at their ends but within them. Slant rhymes are words that are not exact phonemic matches, but still partially or subtly rhyme: compare "white" and "weight" or "sad" and "mad" to "world" and "war," for example.

I will not say quite so much about free verse, except that since William Carlos Williams and then, later, the Beat movement, it has come to dominate our contemporary American poetry scene. Unfortunately, much of the free verse being written today does not explicitly define itself against formal principles, and therefore I think can be devalued; the originators of free verse knew what they were doing, and their disruption of form was precise and deliberate, and lent powerful additional levels of meaning to their work. When we discuss the poems of William Carlos Williams, the distinctions between his work and some of the less accomplished efforts of his many imitators should be apparent.

I would like to focus now, in an introductory fashion, on a few of the poems that I have found most useful in my interactions with patients, specifically four examples that illustrate both the principles by which I have proposed poetry may have a therapeutic effect, and the relevant issues of prosody I have discussed. Of the two poems I will discuss first, one deals with breast cancer and the other with AIDS. Both are written from the perspective of people living with these diseases, either as individual sufferers or as members of an afflicted community.

Marilyn Hacker's seventh book of poems, *Winter Numbers,* was published by W. W. Norton in 1994. One of the most important poets writing in English, she has won numerous literary awards, including the National Book Award and a Guggenheim fellowship; from 1991–94, she edited *The Kenyon Review*, one of the nation's most prestigious and influential literary magazines. A virtuoso of form who was called "our latter-day Byron" by the *New York Times Book Review*, she has courageously taken up themes of relationships between women—feminists, mothers and daughters, and lesbians, whose struggles and pleasures she knows intimately from her own personal experiences. Her diagnosis with breast cancer in 1993 forms the basis for a sequence of sonnets in *Winter Numbers*, from which the poem has been excerpted. Thom Gunn, born in England but a resident of San Francisco since the 1950s, published his *Collected Poems* to wild critical acclaim in 1994; like Marilyn Hacker, he too is considered one of our indispensable poets. His collection *The Man with Night Sweats* was published in 1992 and put a human face on the terrible destruction wrought by the AIDS epidemic. He is a winner of the fabled MacArthur grant and *The Nation*'s Lenore Marshall Poetry Prize. The poem discussed below is reproduced from *The Man with Night Sweats*.

Here is the Hacker sonnet, from a stunning sequence of sonnets entitled "Cancer Winter." I suggest you read the poem aloud now.

> No body stops dreaming it's twenty-five,
> or twelve, or ten, when what is possible's
> a long road poplars curtain against loss, able
> to swim the river, hike the culvert, drive
> through the open portal, find the gold hive
> dripping with liquid sweetness. Risible
> fantasy, if, all the while, invisible
> entropies block the roads, so you arrive
> outside a ruin, where trees bald with blight
> wane by a river drained to sluggish mud.
> The setting sun looks terribly like blood.
> The hovering swarm has nothing to forgive.
> Your voice petitions the indifferent night:
> "I don't know how to die yet. Let me live."[1]

Recalling the principles I have proposed by which poetry may be therapeutic, we find many illustrated here. First note that the poem is written in iambic pentameter, and that the rhyme pattern for most of the poem is abba, cddc, etc. So the poet has chosen a form that immediately establishes her control over the difficult theme of the poem, which attempts to reconcile going on with one's life and the possibly terminal diagnosis of breast cancer. The dream of restored health is contrasted with the prospect of death, and so the entire disease process is deftly captured in the metaphorical constructions of the poem—in the beginning, the able-bodied poet vigorously swims and hikes, her strong, pounding heartbeat clearly audible in the iambic metrical structure, and she sensuously imagines "the gold hive dripping with liquid sweetness;" but her journey, in reality, leads to "a ruin, where trees bald with blight / wane by a river drained to a sluggish mud." The next line, "The setting sun looks terribly like blood" delivers a devastating blow with its end rhyme, the very moment when the poet permits herself to feel and to confront the terrible beauty of death. But the poet never relinquishes her authority, as she is the one insistently telling this story, even though the rhyme scheme is perceptibly altered in the last third of the poem; the poem masterfully culminates in the translocating, urgent, and oddly uplifting plea of the last line: "I don't know how to die yet. Let me live."

Next, read Gunn's poem "The J Car," which further reinforces some of these concepts:

> Last year I used to ride the J CHURCH Line,
> Climbing between small yards recessed with vine
> Their ordered privacy, the plots of flowers
> Like blameless lives we might imagine ours.
> Most trees were cut back, but some brushed the car
> Before it swung round to the street once more
> On which I rolled out almost to the end,
> To 29th Street, calling for my friend.
>   He'd be there, smiling but gaunt,
> To set out for the German restaurant.
> There, since his sight was tattered now, I would
> First read the menu out. He liked the food
> In which a sourness and dark richness meet
> For conflict without taste of a defeat,
> As in the Sauerbraten. What he ate
> I'd hoped would help him to put on some weight,
> But though the crusted pancakes might attract
> They did so more as concept than in fact,
> And I'd eat his dessert before we both
> Rose from the neat arrangement of the cloth,
> Where the connection between life and food
> Had briefly seemed so obvious if so crude.
> Our conversation circumspectly cheerful,

We had sat here like children good but fearful
Who think if they behave everything might
Still against likelihood come out all right.
    But it would not, and we could not stay here:
Finishing up the Optimator beer
I walked him home through the suburban cool
By dimming shape of church and Catholic school,
Only a few white teenagers about.
After the four blocks he would be tired out.
I'd leave him to the feverish sleep ahead,
Myself to ride through darkened yards instead
Back to my health. Of course I simplify.
Of course. It tears me still that he should die
As only an apprentice to his trade,
The ultimate engagements not yet made.
His gifts had been withdrawing one by one
Even before their usefulness was done:
This optic nerve would never be relit;
The other flickered, soon to be with it.
Unready, disappointed, unachieved,
He knew he would not write the much-conceived,
Much-hoped-for work now, nor yet help create
A love he might in full reciprocate.[2]

Again, note the potent effect of the metrical construction and rhyme in animating the poem with the body's natural rhythms. More salient in this example is the clearly nourishing identification with a larger community through illness, so important in other writings in response to AIDS. The poet must actually "read the menu out" for his sight-impaired friend; similarly, one imagines, he is obligated to write about his friend's illness. "The connection between life and food / Had briefly seemed so obvious, if so crude," heartrending in its simplicity, is dramatized in the poet's eating his friend's dessert, as if to sustain his own life through what we come to sense will be an inevitable loss. The poem creates a luminous space for grieving, then, and in its consumption the reader feels in the pit of his own stomach the awful unfulfillment of a life cut short by illness, together with the colorless loneliness of "only a few white teenagers about." A tremendous sense of empathy, which I have found to be powerfully renewing, is created out of the particular details about the dying friend—a young man who, not unlike a medical student or resident at the threshold of a career, has his own talents and trade, and the capacity for love, none of which in this case will reach fruition. The forced understatement of the entire poem is a metaphor itself for this aching disappointment, muted (but not silenced) itself by what stands in starkly ironic contrast as the insatiable epidemic.

The work of many physician-poets also addresses illness and healing, though by no means exclusively, and I believe a consideration of examples of their poetry will further enrich the discussion of some of these points. I will focus briefly on two physician-poets.

Alice Jones is a psychiatrist who practices in Oakland, California. Her first book of poems, *The Knot,* won the 1992 Beatrice Hawley Award and was published by Alice James Books, an innovative cooperative press in Cambridge that specializes in writing by women. Her poems have appeared in numerous magazines, including *Poetry* and *The Kenyon Review.* William Carlos Williams, considered by critics to be the most important literary doctor since Chekhov, died in 1963 after changing contemporary American poetry forever. He published many books of poetry and also many articles on the craft of poetry. He developed the concept of the variable foot, a metrical unit that derived from natural cadences in spoken language. He wrote what some considered "anti-poetry," where the language itself was subverted to the thing, allowing simple details themselves to take on symbolic weight. Though he kept his medical career as a general practitioner in urban New Jersey largely separate from his writing of poetry, many of his poems suggest a keen diagnostic eye and, more important, a deep sense of the human suffering to which he was so often exposed.

Alice Jones's poem "Prayer" can be found below, and like the other poems in this essay, I suggest you read it aloud.

> Send rain, down to the dry bare bones of me,
>   the tarsals planted in sand, no sage
>   or mint or parsley will grow here, snails
>   are sucked dry, leave frail shells
>   in the dug garden's dirt, no flowers, no fronds;
>
> Send rain, down to the deep bowl of my pelvis,
>   barren red hollow, the empty sack
>   sags now with age, the scarred yellow ovals
>   discharge their eggs in irregular cycles,
>   no longer linked so well with the moon;
>
> Send rain, down to the restless quartered meat

that thuds on my ribs, whose valves
measure thin blood as it seeps through
the pipes feeding desiccated organs,
whose mortal work forms sludge;

Send rain, down to the small transparent curve,
the opaque lens that filters dim light
to the lustrous surface and on to dense
convolutions of brain, the task of my sighted
vitreous globes that turn in their padded cells;

Send rain, down to the knots and whorls
where memory continues to pile thick layers,
sloughs surface, and roots reach into
that grey ground where my neurons grow sparse
and leached soil sprouts nothing new.

Send rain.[3]

Though not specifically addressed to a particular illness, this poem none-theless reveals an intimate knowledge of the anatomy of the human body. The incantatory diction places it in unobstructed communication with ancient healers' poetry; its eloquent plea for rain, which the poet imagines may restore the aging body, recalls the Native American view of the suffering individual as part of the larger natural world upon which she depends for wellness. The poet represents the body as open to and available to the elements; here, words themselves become a luxurious rainfall, pouring over us in the long sentence fragments that constitute each stanza. Again, the creation of metaphor—the pelvis becomes a vessel in which to hold rainwater, the orbits become padded cells—carries the reader from one state of being to another, from tired observer to rejuvenated celebrant.

Compare these effects to the William Carlos Williams poem, "The Widow's Lament in Springtime":

Sorrow is my own yard
where the new grass
flames as it has flamed
often before but not
with the cold fire
that closes round me this year.

Thirty-five years
I lived with my husband.
The plumtree is white today
with masses of flowers.
Masses of flowers
loaded the cherry branches
and color some bushes
yellow and some red
but the grief in my heart
is stronger than they
for though they were my joy
formerly, today I noticed them
and turned away forgetting.
Today my son told me
that in the meadows,
at the edge of the heavy woods
in the distance, he saw
trees of white flowers.
I feel that I would like
to go there
and fall into those flowers
and sink into the marsh near them.[4]

In the Williams poem, the characteristic absolutely faithful recording of experience is present, especially at the moment when the phrase "masses of flowers" is repeated, which vividly evokes what the subject of the poem—the widow—is seeing. What is different about this poem, however, is the manner in which the poet also imagines the mind itself. The dissociation of the mind from the physical body is manifest in the conspicuous lack of metrical structure so prominent in the Hacker and Gunn poems, while present in the blank repetition of the poem is the distraction of grieving, as the mind re-records a detail in its preoccupation, too sad to reflect upon the funereal quality of the image, perhaps unconsciously protecting itself from this association. The line break "I lived with my husband. / The plumtree is white today" produces a feeling that is heartrending in its familiarity, as we see the mind deflect itself from some unspoken pain via a non sequitur. Clearly, the overall affect of the poem is depressed, demonstrating the tedious scanning of a world suddenly devoid of emotional resonance in the wake of the loss of a loved one. Remarkably, the poem is not at all overtly sad or, in more extreme terms, sentimental, and to be sure most would argue the avoidance of explicit emotional content is its greatest strength. The poem does not simply evoke the things accessible to a reader by his or her senses but also represents a certain quality of the perceiving mind, of consciousness—even emotion is presented as an object one might come across in the mental landscape. Furthermore, the parallel of the landscape in the poem and the content of the subject's mind is made quite obvious with the powerful opening line "Sorrow is my own yard." In essence, Williams brilliantly catches a human mind in the very act of perceiving. Such insight is crucial to the healing process, a process of renewal that paradoxically is also present in the blooming white flowers of spring.

In this brief essay, I have tried to provide a historical framework for understanding the relationship between poetic expression and a broadly defined concept of healing. I discussed modern bibliotherapy, a vital adjunct to psychiatric care. I proposed several mechanisms by which poetry might have a therapeutic effect on its readers and writers, and after a brief discussion of prosody as the science of poetry, I illustrated by interpreting poems (about each of which much more could be said). I have employed in the care of my own patients some of the healing power of words. I hope that the reader will have reached with me the following conclusions: that, indeed, poetry and healing may be linked; that poetry has basis in the physical body; and that poetry can help educate physicians, as perhaps the inclusion of this essay in this anthology attests. These poems, and many others, should be shared by physicians and patients, and also with medical students and residents.

It seems fitting to end with a quotation from Williams's autobiography, from the short chapter he called "Of Medicine and Poetry," one of his few writings where he considered healing and poetry together. He wrote:

> When they ask me, as of late they frequently do, how I have for so many years continued an equal interest in medicine and the poem, I reply that they amount for me to nearly the same thing. Any worth-his-salt physician knows that no one is "cured." We recover from some somatic, some bodily "fever" where as observers we have seen various engagements between our battalions of cells playing at this or that lethal maneuver with other natural elements. . . . The cured man, I want to say, is no different from any other. It is a trivial business unless you add the zest, whatever that is, to the picture. That's how I came to find writing such a necessity, to relieve me from such a dilemma. I found by practice . . . that to treat a man as something to which surgery, drugs and hoodoo applied was an indifferent matter; to treat him as material for a work of art made him somehow come alive to me.[5]

ENDNOTES

1. Marilyn Hacker, "Cancer Winter," *Winter Numbers* (New York: W. W. Norton, 1994), 77–78.

2. Thom Gunn, "The J Car," *The Man With Night Sweats* (New York: Farrar, Straus and Giroux, 1994), 77.

3. Alice Jones, "The Prayer," *The Knot* (Farmington, Maine: Alice James Books, 1992), 62.

4. Willam Carlos Williams, "The Widow's Lament in Springtime," *Selected Poems* (New York: New Directions Publishing, 1968), 17.

5. William Carlos Williams, *The Autobiography of William Carlos Williams* (New York: New Directions Publishing, 1951), 286, 287.

SECTION TWO

Grand Perspectives

A wonderful gift! How *do*
you find the time for it in

your busy life? It must be a great
thing to have such a pastime.

But you were always a strange
Boy. How's your mother? . . .

Your father was *such* a nice man.
I remember him well.

Or, Geeze, Doc, I guess it's all right.
But what the hell does it mean?
—Paterson, Book 3

Come on!
Do you want to live
forever?—
That
is the essence
of poetry.
But it does not
always
take the same form.
For the most part
it consists
in listening
to the nightingale
or fools.
—"Come on!"

Birth Pangs

F. Gonzalez-Crussi

DOCTOR ERNESTO VIDAL decided early in his career that he would become an obstetrician. Nothing compared, in his estimation, with the awe-inspiring phenomena of human reproduction. The incredible coordination of fetal development, and the dramatic sequences of childbirth, held him in suspension. These prodigies were all around; at the hospital, births could be seen every day, but to him were never commonplace. That a human being should evolve, in the span of a few months, from a mere speck, an invisible particle, into a fully developed organism endowed with heart, eyes, limbs, movement, sentience, and a brain fit to house an individual human consciousness; these were the marvels that, while others grew blasé, Ernesto Vidal continued to consider with unabated amazement.

This is why he remained steadfast in his decision. In his student years, the occasional disparagement from his classmates did not bother him. For it is a fact, well known by those of the profession, that obstetrics is often perceived as lowest in the intellectual scale of the medical specialties. Inside jokes allude to the relatively scant demands for exercise of the reasoning faculty in this field, compared to the rigorous intellectual exactions that, say, internal medicine, wreaks upon its practitioners. "All you are expected to do is to catch the baby," joked the many who supposed there was little need for carefully planned intervention in a process that takes place of its own unstoppable momentum, and has done so since time immemorial. But Vidal's interest did not diminish. He felt it was a privilege and a high honor to attend a normal birth. He was persuaded that criticisms of the "medicalization" of births must recede before the obvious benefits that medical science had brought. The control of pain, the dramatic decrease of puerperal infections, the lower rate of complications, and the improved prospects for the newly born: these conquests could not be denied, even by the harshest critics. They had to admit that scientific advances turned the process of birth into a much less fearful experience for contemporary women than it had been for their grandmothers.

Ernesto Vidal went on to pursue postgraduate training in the United States. It is important to interject here that although our man was a Latin American, his national origin is irrelevant for what followed. The events that took place that day may seem extraordinary, but they are, unfortunately, not at all unusual in a large part of our planet—that vast portion that is euphemistically referred to as "third world," and which constitutes, by far, its largest and most populous fraction. Here, back in his own country, Doctor Vidal was in daily contact with the complications of pregnancy. The birth of babies in conditions of dismal poverty and hopelessness was habitual in his practice.

Now, those who witness a child with the harrowing stigmata of malnutrition even as it emerges from its mother's womb, doomed to learning disabilities on account of impaired brain development, and released to ignorant parents who live in insalubrious, depressing circumstances, can hardly repress a pessimist outlook. To see an innocent child, just born, yet already hindered by manifold dysfunctions, is nothing less than depressing. To see, then, the frail infant turned over to ignorant care takers in a crime-ridden, stultifying environment, inevitably evokes the famous Sophoclean lines in *Oedipus at Colonnus:* "The best were not to be born at all, / But once born, the next best thing is to return immediately to where one came from."

It is a tribute to Doctor Vidal's resilience (some might say a token of his naiveté and misjudgment) that such dark thoughts never crossed his mind. Others became jaded, or insensitive. But somehow he managed to preserve what one may call, for lack of a better word, enthusiasm. This was a unique sentiment, a mixture of indescribable tenderness and wonder that invaded him upon witnessing a new birth. Many a terrible complication was averted through his expertise. But, had he attended normal births only, he never would have felt that his job was routine. For he never lost the feeling that what he was doing was something important. He was the minister of a life ritual of uncommon significance; the diapason vibrating in unison with a mighty life-wave that stirred, indomitable, over the whole world. In every birth he saw something forceful, affirmative, unalterably confident. Be it natural optimism or plain misreckoning, his turn of mind made him detect a positive accent in the cry of the countless children he brought into the light.

Unwavering enthusiasm for his work was one of the elements of his success. He aspired to an academic career, and obtained a position at the Women's Hospital, his country's largest, and one of the biggest of its kind in the world. It was a matter of pride for him that, while still relatively young, his post was one of considerable responsibility. In the afternoon shift, the most experienced professors being absent, Ernesto Vidal was in charge of an entire ward with dozens of patients. The hospital was within the university campus, his own alma mater. From the window of his ward, one could see the building where he had studied biology as an undergraduate. Across the street, also clearly within view from the window, was the School of Philosophy, an old building with pretentious decorations that flaunted on its facade a row of niche-like recesses harboring the marble busts or life-sized statues of illustrious thinkers, ancient and modern.

One afternoon, as he readied himself to drive to the hospital, his wife called his attention to the news on the radio. There was unrest in the streets. The students had been manifesting a little too vociferously. The "forces of the constituted order," pompously said the news report, were forced to confront them. In short, the government had warned the protesters that they would be repressed with little regard for the consequences. "Be careful, Ernesto," said his wife, "why don't you wait here to see what develops?" But this admonition, voiced in a lukewarm tone, was all she advanced by way of warning. As a woman, she was fully cognizant of the kind of womanly suffering that her husband made it his calling to alleviate. She did not insist, except by reiterating her strong urging to be very, very careful. Ernesto Vidal assured her there was no reason to worry, kissed her on the cheek, got into his car, and drove away.

In the expressway leading to the campus, the traffic slowed down. He was listening to the radio when the flow of cars came to a complete stop. The police deployed its forces, soon the university campus would be completely encircled, and it would be difficult to reach his destination. The line of cars ahead of him seemed interminable. He stepped out of his vehicle, and joined the small group of impatient drivers who had done the same thing, and who now chatted among themselves, or vented their frustration with sundry expressions of discontent.

"I've been trying to get to my office for the last hour and a half! Usually, I can make it in twenty minutes," said one of the stranded commuters.

"Those stupid brats!" exclaimed another. "They don't have to earn a living, as do their parents. It is high time the authorities should make them toe the line, once and for all!" But this expression of fierce conservatism met the reproof of other stranded drivers, who maintained that the students had legitimate grievances, and lay the blame for the troubles at the door of the government.

It seemed that a discussion was beginning to shape itself, when a crackling noise occurred in the distance, followed by the roar of an invisible multitude. It did not require much experience to guess that it was the noise of gunfire, echoed by the indistinct screams of a faraway crowd. The stranded drivers fell silent and looked at each other in consternation. At that very moment, however, the circulation was restarted, and they returned to their cars.

Ernesto Vidal left the expressway at the first opportunity, convinced that, everything considered, he would save time if he tried to reach the hospital through back streets. But he found many streets already cordoned off by the police, and was forced to follow a very circuitous route. He turned into a strangely deserted alley, perceived that some activity was taking place at the end of it, which he took to be road repairs, and pressed on, in utter disregard of the directional signs that indicated he was advancing against the permitted sense. Midway down the alley he realized a group of students comprised the group he had mistaken for repairmen. They were raising a barricade. He was approached by some, and, after identifying himself, he was allowed to go through. Not without first being asked to contribute some money to their cause.

"It is to buy guns to defend ourselves," one of their number matter-of-factly volunteered.

To which Doctor Vidal replied, collectedly: "I sympathize with your cause. But I don't think I would be helping you if I gave you money for that purpose. You can take the box of medicaments I have in the trunk of my car. Or one of you can come with me to the hospital, where I promise to give you a whole load of bandages, wound disinfectants, and first aid kits that you may be needing. But I won't contribute money for guns. I will give you nothing that might increase the bloodshed."

The student's angry retort was: "In the first place, sir, it is not *our* cause, as you so complacently put it. It is yours as much as it is ours. And it is nice of you to sound so sanctimonious and to preach nonviolence, but I don't much appreciate your kind of smugness . . ."

A gleam of wrath shone in his eyes as he said this, but he was promptly interrupted by one of his comrades, who grabbed him by the arm and said, while pulling him away from Vidal's car window: "Let him go, friend. Let him go. Don't lose your time with this man. You can see that he is thoroughly brainwashed . . ."

The group of students made way for his vehicle, and Vidal did not tarry. He pressed the accelerator, and soon was in the avenue that led to the hospital. As he reached his destination, and parked his car, he could not avoid thinking of this encounter. Was he, as the student had opined, "thoroughly brainwashed"? The students were right in protesting. This much he knew. The government was irredeemably corrupt. Social injustices were all too glaring. But only the young had the courage to say this loudly. When young, he, too, had protested. He, too, had been a student, marched in demonstrations, carried placards, and confronted the police. Now he tended to regard all that as transient, youthful thoughtlessness. Most of all, it was useless. After mature deliberation, he had concluded that the protests in the streets were ineffective. There were public disturbances, a few broken skulls, perhaps even some deaths, headlines in the newspapers for a week; and then, nothing. No: his duty was to be a good physician and a good teacher. Everyone had to do his job to the best of his or her ability. This, in effect, was the answer to much of the distemper that afflicted society.

But this way, presently he reflected, change was not any more apt to come by. He had done his best to excel at his job. And his achievement had been recognized. His was a position of responsibility, well remunerated, and generally respected. Although not rich, he lived a comfortable life, and his wife and children enjoyed the amenities of the middle class. Was not the fear of compromising all that, the real reason for his conformity? The young did not have much to lose; but he had many things to worry about: his position in society, his status as a member of the medical profession, the welfare of his family, the future of his children. And as he thought of all this, he could not suppress the melancholy feeling that the student who inveighed on his passivity was correct. The practice of medicine had taught him firsthand that the roots of many of the ills he surveyed were out of his reach. Infant mortality, teen pregnancy, venereal infections, developmental defects: these and many other ailments derived ultimately from ignorance, poverty, and society's callous indifference. And those in whose power it was to alleviate these ills cared about nothing but their own increscent wealth. *Someone* had to sound a loud, urgent, unwavering protest. But, of course, this someone would not be himself. The student had been right. He, Doctor Ernesto Vidal, would end by soothing his scruples in the smug proclamation that everyone had an appointed job; that he was a physician, with no time for any other endeavor than the care of the sick; and that as long as he fulfilled this duty, there would be a God in heaven, and all would be well with the world.

This was his train of thought when he finally came to the hospital, and hurried through the corridors. It was close to two hours later than his habitual check-in time when he donned his hospital coat. No sooner had he done this, than he was called to the emergency room. A woman, picked up unconscious from a grimy, miserable bedroom, her forehead covered with a cold sweat, in a state of shock, had just been brought in by ambulance. A neighbor declared that the patient had undergone an abortion, probably performed in dismal conditions of hygiene.

"I suspect the neighbor herself had something to do with the misdeed," said one of the paramedics. "She is the one who called us."

Doctor Vidal had no time to waste. He was soon drawn into the maelstrom of activity that was customary. He ordered blood tests, intravenous infusions, antibiotics, and medicaments that would raise the patient's dangerously low blood pressure. Then, he went up to the fourth floor, to the ward that was directly under his care. He had not been there more than five minutes, when he noted a commotion at the end of the corridor.

There, he found nurses, orderlies, and students congregated by a window that looked to the north of the campus. They were quite agitated, had opened

wide the window's casements, and shouted excitedly. The reason for this flur-
ried discomposure was outside. A large group of students had come running,
in a confused scatter, generally in the direction of the university buildings
closest to the hospital. Evidently they were desperate for shelter, as they were
being persecuted by uniformed, riot-control policemen. Those who did not
run or were intercepted by the police were mercilessly beaten. And the spectacle of unarmed youths being decimated by well-trained, gun-toting, club-
wielding, organized force, angered beyond measure the hospital employees
who watched the action from the window. "To the right! To the right!" they
screamed, trying to orient the youngsters who eluded capture. "Don't let them
get you!" "For God's sake, run! Run!" At the same time, some shouted insults
at the persecuting policemen: "Bastards!" "Bullies!" and other niceties that
would have made the vilest rabble blush.

It took Doctor Vidal no small effort to calm down the watchers and per-
suade them to go back to their duties.

"Doctor Vidal, don't you have blood in your veins? Can't you see what
those bastards are doing to the students?" said a nurse, reproachfully.

"I see it, and I am as disgusted as any of you. I sympathize with those kids.
The university is my own alma mater, and I hate to see this violence taking
place on its grounds. But our first obligation is to our patients. Remember that.
You cannot simply abandon the patients under your care, not on account of
what is happening outside. If it were a full-blown revolution, your first duty
still lies with your patients, who need your help."

This appeal was especially effective. There were, indeed, plenty of patients
needing immediate care. Defenseless women whose lives, and those of their
children, depended—literally—on appropriate, promptly administered treatment. The hospital workers returned to their posts, but in the hours that followed their activities were periodically interrupted by episodes of window
watching accompanied by emotional outbursts. Outside, there were skirmishes
between the rebellious students and the guardians of law and order. Inside,
the millenarian, intense hand-to-hand combat between mother and child un-
folded, now rapidly and with a felicitous outcome, now laboriously and under
the ominous sign of deadly complications.

A large contingent of students had reached the building of the School of
Philosophy, and from its roof, or from its windows, hurled stones at their
besiegers. This could not be seen easily from the patients area, but some patients had wandered to the corridor, and those not well enough to get up
from bed knew intuitively what was occurring, or conjectured it from what
they heard. A number of women were in labor, and the course of their delivery seemed adversely affected by the tension and disquietude that reigned

outside. For the patients, in their distress, troubled by the noises and the alarms of the staff, naturally concurred in the idea that it was a sad thing to give birth to a child in the midst of these inauspicious developments.

"I thought this would be a light day," commented a resident physician. "With the streets blocked all around us, I assumed the patients were going to be taken to other hospitals and clinics."

"No such luck, my friend," replied one of his comrades. "The ambulances are being let through."

This was true. Ambulances and other conveyances carrying patients were usually not allowed to cross police lines. Vidal wondered if the police force, inexplicably benevolent, had yielded this time to medical urgency out of humane compassion.

The resident's comment he deemed closer to the truth: "You know, a conspicuously pregnant woman with a big belly sends a message of great urgency. Men, especially, hate to have to deal with this kind of problem. Mostly they fear it. They fear the imminence, the not being in control, and the irrevocability of childbirth. Rather than to have a messy, bloody, little wriggler on their lap, they would let the car go through, right away, without stopping to argue with the driver, and then put it all down to their enlightened compassion."

Doctor Vidal is now summoned to see a patient. In the corridors, wearing hospital gowns and slippers, or from their beds, the patients question him anxiously: "What is happening?" "Is the hospital safe?" "Are we going to be all right?" Vidal reassures them. Not to worry, everything is under control. The outside disturbance will soon be over.

He reaches the bed of the patient he was called to see. She is a young girl, probably thirteen or fourteen years old. She is intensely pale, and looks around with the big, brown, liquid eyes of a frightened gazelle. Vidal is told that "she is not progressing," that is, her labor has been inordinately prolonged. Then, he hears a confusing history of ill-advised obstetrical intervention. She was told in some disreputable slum clinic (exactly where, she cannot or will not say) that her child "was coming in the wrong position." A maneuver was attempted to correct the malposition. But, clearly, the maneuver was unnecessarily rough, performed by ignorant and inexperienced operators, and may have caused grave harm. There is the possibility of rupture of the uterus, although this diagnosis is not certain. The status of the fetus also needs more careful evaluation. Vidal requests X-ray films, and indicates to the resident the dispositions to be taken.

He asks the girl whether her husband is with her. She replies that she has no husband. Her boyfriend? The girl turns aside, toward the wall, without answering.

"Please tell us, it is important," adds Doctor Vidal. "Is your boyfriend the father of your baby?" But the girl remains silent.

A resident adds: "The man who brought her here came with his wife. They were a middle-aged couple who said they were friends of her family. They left in a hurry, before anyone could have questioned them in more detail."

"Did they tell you what was done at the outside clinic?"

"They said a doctor told them that they had tried to 'straighten out' the baby, but she did not stand the procedure well. And then, when things started to turn sour, they advised them to bring the patient here immediately. Or else, they pointed out, they would not be responsible for what happened to her."

"Ah yes . . ." Doctor Vidal retorted laconically. How many times had he heard that sort of story? A blunder, a well-nigh criminal misdeed, and then the precipitous, frantic efforts to deny all responsibility. Ship the patient out! Take her to the tertiary-care center, immediately. You must do this straight away, or else you—not us—must bear the entire responsibility for the consequences.

Vidal is about to leave the room when, unexpectedly, the child-mother addresses him. Hesitatingly, as if crushed under a big weight, she says: "The father of my baby is my stepfather."

Ernesto Vidal is momentarily disconcerted. He has heard many heart-rending stories of misery and despair. But he cannot help recoiling upon hearing this sudden, grievous declaration. What abysses of poverty, promiscuity and abjection lurk behind this girl's—this child's—avowal? This is something that he cannot fathom. Once more, his thoughts turn to his own powerlessness. The real causes of the evil he is forced to face fall outside his purview. True, he will repair the lacerations, and will treat the infections as well as possible. Yet, he cannot delude himself any longer: behind wounds and infections lies a violent, prepotent energy that shall continue to tear women's wombs and fester their hearts: the evil force of ignorance, superstition, and sheer human cruelty.

At the same time, a profound pity, an immense tenderness wells up in the depth of his being for this poor, defenseless child-mother. It is an overmastering feeling that he does not know how to express with words. He places his hand lovingly on the girl's forehead and tells her: "Do not worry. You and your child are going to be all right. We are going to do all we can for you. I promise you that."

Outside, the students have fortified themselves inside the buildings of the university. Doors are barricaded by tables and various objects thrown across them. Obstacles have been erected in passages to check the advance of the besiegers. The besiegers, on the other hand, have skillfully mobilized their forces. Many men are now posted on the roof of neighboring buildings. Immobile, reclining against ledges and parapets, a posse of sharpshooters points its weapons at the School of Philosophy, the redoubt of most of the rebels. It seems as if a firing squad is getting ready to execute a row of marble philosophers who frown and adopt heroic poses in their niches, on the building's facade.

The chief of police arrives carrying a portable loudspeaker and summons the entrenched students to surrender, using words that seem copied from a Hollywood gangster film: "Come out with your hands up!" To which the students reply with insults and hurled stones. Once again, nurses and other personnel are at the window, unable to contain their wrath, and direct rounds of vituperation at the police. The noise of all this tumult is well heard in the area of the patients, and some of them begin to cry. Those who can, stand up from their beds and attempt to come to the window. This forces Doctor Vidal to take stronger measures. He orders the patients back to their beds, all the windows closed shut, and all the curtains drawn.

The area now becomes somewhat hot and stuffy. Vidal refuses several petitions to reopen the windows. "Hold on a little longer," he says. And as he visits the child-mother and finds out that a rupture of the uterus has been ruled out, though her labor contractions have become less frequent with the passage of time, he cannot avoid the suspicion that the outward circumstances and their psychological impact may be an important factor that inhibits the delivery. But he cannot linger in this sort of speculation. A colleague comes to tell him that the patient he first saw upon coming to the hospital, the woman with the septic abortion, is now getting worse and will be transported to the intensive care unit. A team of specialists in critical care medicine is looking after her. For some time, Doctor Vidal will be relieved of this problem.

An unscientific mind may have invoked influences other than psychological as a cause of the excessive delay in the labor and delivery of the patients in Doctor Vidal's ward. An irrational belief posits a mysterious "sympathy" between the progress of the fetus in the birth canal, and the obstacles that encumber the mother's surroundings. Thus, in rural Russia, the walls of the house where a woman is in travail display icons, and all the locks in every part of the property must be opened; and all the knots must be untied; and even the plaited blond pigtails of the rosy-cheeked peasant girls who have come to assist with the house chores must be loosened. There must be nothing that may conjure the idea of tightness or union. Parturition requires openness, freedom from encumbrance; this is the time of disunion, or separation of what was formerly bound together.

There are parts of the Muslim world in which the symbolism is still more direct. The tradition there is that not only doors and windows should be open, but the doors of the nearest mosque are also open, and the woman in labor carries an amulet in which are inscribed the first four sentences of the eighty-fourth Sutra of the Koran, which is suggestively entitled "The Splitting Asunder."

Inside the hospital, there was no freedom, no clearance, and no openness: the women's bodies had become traps for the unborn. Everywhere there was tension, anxiety, contraction, and blockade. Ernesto Vidal reflected, perhaps for the first time in his life, that it may have been better thus. He thought: "If a child does not want to be born now, who would blame it?"

He was distracted from his musing by a renewed din outside. The forces of law and order began a well organized assault toward the building where most of the students were entrenched, the School of Philosophy. Incredibly, the students successfully repulsed them. They threw stones, firecrackers (was it really firecrackers?), bricks, and whatever objects could be made into missiles, at the police, who, discountenanced by the fierceness of the resistance, were forced to retreat. Vidal thought, upon hearing the explosions and commotion, of the student who had asked him for money to buy guns.

It is perhaps an idle reflection, but it is one that obtruded itself in the mind at the time: the struggles that were taking place inside and outside the hospital shared some similarities. In both places two opposite, irreconcilable tendencies met one another. In both areas, a desperate eviction effort clashed against a stubborn resistance to dislodgment. Inside, Doctor Vidal was saying: "This baby will not come out, and all the signs are that he is not well. We cannot wait any longer. We'd better prepare the mother for surgery, we must go after that baby, before it is too late." Outside, the chief of police was shouting through the loudspeaker: "All of you, come out! Come out with your hands up!" To which injunction the besieged answered "Cowards! Assassins! Pigs! Come and get us!"

Would that persuasion had worked in either situation! But the opposing parties heard no arguments. Rebellious, exasperated youths will not yield to words of an arbitrary power they despise and have united themselves to oppose. And poorly educated, ill-paid policemen will not debate with youths they have long been taught to consider privileged, poltroon, and unpatriotic. A physiologically inert uterus will not expel a fetus, and the latter will not come out of its own volition. Only in imagination does the fetus work out its own release. In the folklore of many countries, the curious idea survives that the fetus may be enticed or encouraged to quit its cell. Persian midwives placed before the birthing mother toys, pretty infant's clothes, or other objects that might incite the baby to come out, and during labor called: "Come, child, come!" In Egypt, a child was made to play, hop, or dance between the laboring mother's legs, so that the unborn should be taken with the desire to come out and play. And in the Dutch Indies, the father placed himself between the outspread legs of the parturient woman and ran away, presumably in order that the unborn child should wish to imitate his father, and run out himself.

Soon after Doctor Vidal had given the order that the young girl should be taken to the operating room, an ominous rumor spread through the ward. "Soldiers are coming! They are bringing the army!" someone exclaimed. Despite the prohibition, everyone ran to the windows, balconies, or any other available observation post. Suddenly, every gaze was concentrated on the same bend of the main avenue, the turn that led to the campus, and on which military vehicles came rumbling in orderly formation.

"Look, there they are! Tanks! My God, they are bringing tanks!" exclaimed the watchers.

The remark was inaccurate. The vehicles were not tanks, but armored cars, whose heavy, lateral steel plates, furnished with fat rivets and surmounted by a little turret, made them resemble tanks. A helmeted trooper, visible only from the waist up, emerged from the turret behind an impressive machine gun that looked like a little cannon. Behind these forbidding war engines, there were several military trucks that stopped with a screech in front of the School of Philosophy and disgorged their cargo of uniformed men. With the perfectly executed, precise motions of professional soldiers, the men jumped out of the truck and deployed themselves in formation, as if this maneuver had been carefully rehearsed many times before.

None of this was seen by Ernesto Vidal, for at that very minute he was bending over the sedated child-mother, whose frail body was covered by green sterile sheets under the intense glare of the operating room's lamps, to whisper to her some words of comfort. Drowsy, she lifted her large, liquid eyes— eyes of wild game under pursuit— toward the voice, but did not immediately recognize Ernesto Vidal behind the surgical mask that covered his face. Shortly thereafter, her gaze transmitted some sort of ineffable gratitude, just as the anesthesiologist pushed the plunger of a syringe, and she fell into a deep, dark well, or was projected into a long tunnel of muffled echoes and receding, blurring sights, a narrow passage that pulled her ever deeper into darkness and into total unconsciousness.

At the window, the ward personnel looked outside. They could hardly give credit to their eyes, that such a formidable force would be used to overwhelm a group of pugnacious, discontented youths. But it was true. Oppressive governments have long done this, whether in China's Tiananmen Square or in Mexico City's Tlatelolco Square. Was it not true that even in the United States of America, National Guardsmen shot and killed unarmed, defenseless students who protested the Vietnam War at Kent State University?

A student's voice was heard haranguing the soldiers: "Why do you shoot at us? We are not criminals. We are your own compatriots, your neighbors, your brothers, your sons. Your duty is to defend the country from enemy aggression. In God's name, stop and think: We are not the enemy! What lies are your generals telling you to turn you into murderers? How much do they pay you?" But this speech had little effect on a group of men who were raised in poverty, and were rescued from destitution by the army. In Doctor Vidal's country, the army recruits were peasants who tilled an ungrateful land, and who might have starved, had it not been for the army. The army had given them a sense of personal dignity. The army had restored to them and their families a measure of pride. Their allegiance was to the army, and this was not going to change on account of the half-cooked dialectic of a cornered, frightened, middle-class university student.

In the operating room, Ernesto Vidal had barely traced one-half of the incision on the abdominal skin of the child-mother; rivulets of blood were still running, like crimson springs surging forth from a furrow in a fatty glebe that the sharp, stainless-steel plow had just opened; when the rattling, repetitive sound of a machine gun was heard, echoed by the resounding, mighty crash of broken glass. The two surgeons stopped, as if frozen, for only three or four seconds. They looked at each other in bewilderment, their puzzlement concentrated in their eyes, all the more intense for being the only part of their visages that the surgical attire left exposed between the face mask and the head cover. Then, without saying a word, as if their gaze had been sufficient to agree on a strategy, they renewed their surgical work. The operation proceeded, as if nothing had happened.

Outside, the final assault had begun. The machine-gunning of a large window, in one of the upper stories of the building that housed the School of Philosophy, was the starting signal. Later, the military commander of the operation was going to declare to the press that his intelligence had assured him that there were no students behind that window, but at the time this was by no means clear. The spectators of this action were horrified. Except for the personnel devoted to emergencies or currently engaged in critical activities, such as the work taking place in the operating rooms, almost every member of the hospital staff had run to position themselves in an observation post. The watchers were aghast. Everyone believed that a massacre was taking place, and could scarcely give credit to their own eyes. It surpassed all credibility, that a civilized, modern state would employ the technology of advanced warfare to mow down a group of young university students.

A massacre was not the word for what taking place, but a cruel, repressive action it was, nonetheless. And it was carried out with unmitigated savagery.

The police and the army detachments coordinated their respective movements, to flush out the students. After the machine gun shattered the window, the students retreated, and the invaders used ropes and scales to occupy the vacated space. A swift, relentless wave of uniformed men came upon the rebels from all sides. The hospital workers saw the corridors, windows, and alleys of the campus crawling with armed men, who kept pushing forward, relentlessly. Groups of students were caught between the forces of the assailants, as if between the two arms of a pair of pincers. They retreated before the well-armed soldiers with bayonets at the ready, and fell prey to the club-wielding police. The formerly cohesive groups now dispersed in the confusion of the melee. Resistance weakened appreciably as the invaders gained ground.

Some youngsters put up a gallant fight, only to fall to the ground beneath a hail of stick blows. Others, in a show of bravery that was vociferously cheered by onlookers from the hospital, made a sally to assist their fallen comrades, and suffered the same fate. All of this was happening amidst a thunderous roar made by the cries of anger of the attackers, the moaning of the wounded, the noise of glass being broken and of objects hurled at each other, and the screams, oaths, and insults of the contending groups, mixed with the unrestrained exclamations of the witnesses by the windows. All were captured, systematically, and rarely without beatings. The prisoners were thrown into military trucks and whisked away, nobody knew where. Those hurt or unconscious—dead some of them? How many? No one could tell—together with their seemingly uninjured or less seriously wounded confederates.

While the last student was brought out of the School of Philosophy, dragged by the hair, a few meters away from there, in the operating room, Ernesto Vidal was pulling a newly born child out of his mother's womb. With great care he took hold of the slippery, wriggling limbs of the infant, still daubed with whitish sebum, the *vernix caseosa*, and reddish streaks of blood, and deposited it on the green sheets under the lamps of the operating room.

As he aspirated the secretions of the infant's throat with a rubber pump, he asked himself what all this meant. What did it mean to bring one child into the world in the same parcel of space, and in the same division of time, where men mangled, bruised, beat, and perhaps killed each other mercilessly and inhumanely? He knew that there was no rational answer. All he could sense—it was more an obscure intuition than a clear idea—was that all of us, human beings, are the playthings of contrary forces—birth and death, generation and annihilation—without any concern for our individuality. Nature, he thought, does not really care for us as individuals. She is not perturbed by killings or hecatombs. Nature is never aggrieved: *Natura non contristatur*, said the ancients. She keeps on going in her ceaseless, sempiternal, dual rhythms of germination and destruction, quite unmindful of our nice little concepts about the precious and irreplaceable nature of each human being.

It was dawn when he was getting ready to leave the ward and go back home. The last patient he saw was the child-mother, still groggy from sedation and post-anesthesia effects. She could barely articulate a few words of gratitude, to which Doctor Vidal replied: "Don't worry. Rest well. It is a fine looking boy! The two of you are going to be all right." He pressed her hand as he told her these words, and felt that her hand returned, weakly, the friendly grip.

He did not tell her that he harbored doubts about the well being of the baby. The trauma he suffered before birth could have caused some damage. But this was not certain: neurological examination is notoriously difficult in infants. It may be necessary to wait months, or years, to see whether the child met the appropriate developmental milestones in a timely fashion. It was inappropriate to express doubts and reservations at this moment. And then, it was not certain that deficits would ensue. Babies had this uncanny capacity to regenerate damaged tissue; to outgrow the damage; to heal dire lesions against insurmountable odds. Life has a mighty energy to oppose the forces of destruction. And this, he understood, was what kept him from falling into irredeemable cynicism or heartless skepticism. He was on the side of life.

He left his hospital gown in his locker, and looked through the window. The sun had spread a crimson tint admixed with gold on the sky. The ground was littered with the debris of the pitched battle that had been waged hours before. A few police guards had remained on site, and barred the passage. The silence of the place, and the littered, deserted grounds, recalled to Doctor Vidal's mind what had taken place. Here, the uproar of the tumult, the noise of broken glass, the cries of pain of the wounded, the horrified screams, the oaths of the combatants, and the slow-flowing streams of blood on the floor, winding their way around the cobblestones. And there, close by, behind a wall, just a few yards away from this scene, were women who strained, and moaned, and invoked the celestial powers to help them bring their children into the world. And he had been there all the time, amidst the women who sweat and strain, and put forth babies who writhe on the sheets, their little bodies covered with silvery sebum and streaked with blood.

Ernesto Vidal took a deep breath and thought: "This is what I am. I am a tool of the creative force, call it what you will. Others will continue to massacre and exterminate, in the name of ideology or high-sounding shibboleths. They are the ministers of destruction. But I shall be here, on the side of life. This is my job, and this is what I am." He lifted his eyes toward the School of Philosophy, its facade now scarred by the impact of bullets or stones. He could discern the bust of Schopenhauer amidst the effigies of others whose identities he did not know. Ernesto Vidal wondered: "What would the great man think about all this?" He looked at the statue, as if he expected an answer from it. But Schopenhauer looked straight ahead, past him, aloof and unconcerned. He had the same look the night before, by the flickering light of the Molotov cocktails, amidst the diffusing volutes of the tear-gas bombs. The great thinker was absorbed in meditation, imperturbable, looking straight ahead with his marble eyes without pupils.

What, in effect, did the great man think about all that? Perhaps he reflected on the insignificance of individual human life, and the mighty, eternal struggle of the human species.

Mercy Shall Follow

SUSAN ONTHANK MATES

I cannot say of any condition of human life, "This is fixed, this is clearly good, or bad."

—SOPHOCLES, *ANTIGONE*

IN PAIN THEY incarnate, the women of the public wards, and in pain their daughters return. We, the staff, shave and prep and enema and scrub, and God knows deliver when the doctors are too busy, even though some of us are only LPNS. It's amazing we noticed women's lib at all, cratered as our days are with pill counts, notes, sign-overs, waiting in the dusk for the Five train, drafted sons, husbands, dishes, the scramble of what must be done. So many of us come from Jamaica, or Liberia, or the Philippines, it's hard to even see those Westchester girls with all their parents' money and their effortless educations. And yet.

Dr. Brown stands, as he always does, and we respect him for it, in front of the new students and questions. He's a tough one, he is, taking on Hitler, saving people, surviving. We admire his dedication to the babies, to life. We're afraid of the head-on crash between him and the girl, each so sure of themselves. But at the end of the day, what's it to us? Their lives aren't ours. They work here and go home somewhere else, somewhere that smells of grass and woods and money.

The door to Dr. Brown's office rests open; we glance sometimes, bringing a chart, a report, at the walls hung with diplomas. And over the desk, gilt-edged:

ד' רֹעִי, לֹא אֶחְסָר.

The Lord is my shepherd; I shall not want.

His family wasn't religious; the first time he heard a Psalm was in a foxhole, fighting for the Resistance. Brown tells the story and laughs; while the guy was praying, Brown was on the other side of the trench, with a woman, doing something else. Each time we hear it, we smile to be polite, each time, when he leaves, we groan and roll our eyes.

"I don't know what's complaining louder, my feet or my back," says the girl on Days from Four South, "You got any aspirin in that bag of yours?" She's thick and short, from Manila, and her English sounds like Tagalog.

"I saw the libber girl yesterday, you see her?" Four South Evenings says, still sweating from the heat of the stairs and rummaging in her vinyl handbag. "Wearing that loud miniskirt and those platforms waving her little butt in the air," Evenings is tall and skinny and holds herself very straight. She came from Ivory Coast as a teenager. She pulls out a squat bottle and hands it to Days.

"It's a bad idea, taking those kids on the wards right away. Poor things, they dart around like scared chickens. And with Dr. Brown of all people. Want to start with room five or twenty-seven? Anybody unstable?" Days pops down two pills with the flat remainder of a Coke, gives the bottle back to Evenings with a nod, and lights up a cigarette. She relaxes a little and thinks about whether the train will be on time, what she's going to make for dinner, and whether her son will be home like he said he would. "The girl's name is MacKenzie, made a point of introducing herself. Looks like trouble. I'll promise you this, *she's* got no one depending on her—no kids, no man, no sick old mom. Things look different from that point of view." Days laughs. Evenings does not.

We're signing over shifts when we see them, the students running through the ward, nervous and chattering. The boys bang open the fire door and crash down the stairs to the cafeteria, but the girl, Mackie, pulls over the older girl, Lucille.

"That's the one with a kid?" whispers the ward secretary to Four South Evenings, rolling her eyes toward Lucille. "How does she think she's going to do it?"

"Lucille," Mackie says, grabbing her by the arm, pulling her away from the nurses' station and into an alcove, "we've got to do something. We didn't get here just to be as bad as *they* are."

Lucille is taller than Mackie; her face is quiet and broad. Mackie's slight and pale, with red-blond hair floating around her face. Lucille squints at Mackie's fierce expression. "What are you talking about?"

"You're shaking, Lucille, don't tell me it doesn't bother you. Don't tell me he wasn't trying to torture you by asking all those questions right in front of that poor naked lady having her baby and ignoring her. Don't tell me he didn't pick on you because you'd feel it the worst, identify with her."

Lucille sighs. "The point, Mackie?" Lucille looks away at the peeling green paint on the door to the utility room. A fly buzzes past. "Don't get me wrong," she says, almost angrily, "I know you jumped in to distract him from me."

Mackie leans forward and says, "I'm going to stop him using those women. Did they volunteer to have a bunch of strangers learn about female genitalia on their naked bodies while they lie there helpless?"

"We have to learn somehow," says Lucille. "Otherwise, there wouldn't be any doctors." She smoothes her skirt. "And, besides, we're just students. We might get in the way of the deliveries."

"Don't Catholics believe 'Blessed is he that considereth the poor'?" She looks at Lucille with a small, ironic, smile.

Lucille is silent for a moment. "Mackie," she says, in a hard voice, "I rode the subway to take night school organic chemistry, standing, every day of my pregnancy. And my religion is none of your business." She turns away from Mackie and starts to leave.

Mackie raises her chin and looks at her. "You want to know my religion? We hold these truths to be self-evident, that all men are created equal, that they are endowed by their Creator with certain unalienable Rights." Mackie looks calm but the veins stand out on her neck. "Do men have to lie on their backs with their legs spread, naked, while women stand around and look at them, ignore their pain, shove things into them, and call it teaching?"

"I don't agree," says Lucille. "Rules are for the patients' own good, so they can get to you fast, if they need to. You wouldn't understand. You've never had a child yourself—the mothers want the baby safe, even if it means they give up a little privacy."

"It's not necessary to treat them like animals. I'll hand out my pamphlets, you do whatever you want."

"You're so arrogant, Mackie, with that WASP noblesse oblige." Lucille watches Mackie's face and sees the slight shift in the set of her lips, the hurt. "Look, I couldn't have dealt, the way you did, with your father. And then your mother, when you were just a kid. But don't do this, Mackie. Listen to me: I'm older than you. Things aren't so simple."

"Right and wrong are simple."

Lucille shrugs her shoulders. "I've got a husband and a daughter, I want to be a doctor," she says, "that's simple." She pushes open the stairwell door that leads down to the cafeteria, where the rest of the group is waiting.

Four months earlier, Dr. Brown strides across the roads and lawns from Women's Hospital to the Medical School. The little grasses of spring, he thinks, stab through an unwilling slush. He watches a web of clouds drift across the sun and feels the intrusion of memory. Buttoning up his white coat, he enters the low concrete building, takes the stairs two at a time, and walks into the conference room, last one there. The admissions' meeting has already begun.

The black-browed hematologist-turned-biochemist says, "I only care about their grades and board scores. Let them be white, black, purple, male, female, hermaphrodite, just give me smart and hard-working."

The practicing pediatrician from Long Island says, "But Jack, the women take up slots and then quit to get married and raise kids. Sandy agrees."

They turn and look at Dr. Brown who responds with a small look of distaste. He shrugs his shoulders. "The Dean," he says, "knows my opinion of women."

The administrator says, "I don't know about you, Fred, but I'd rather a B student with maturity and compassion take care of me than an A student-psychopath." The others continue as if he hadn't spoken.

Several agree to take a few women, as long as they are top students. It helps attract the better men. There's a girl, Louise MacKenzie, they all rate high: summa MIT, honors in physics and philosophy. But only one person argues for Lucille Peltier, the married twenty-eight-year-old with a kid.

"Look," says the psychiatrist, "she took the MCATs three times and got better each time, even if the overall score wasn't great. That shows determination."

And, think the others, that shows that she's likely to be even less of a credit to the school than you are, but they vote "yes," anyway, just to shut him up. By the time the class is filled, the sun beats the pavement like a tinsmith, corrugating sidewalks with shimmering heat. Summer erupts.

We hover over our paper-cup coffee, we smash out our cigarettes. On these hot days, it's best to start before the sun. We sigh and get going. Out in the hall, Dr. Brown yells at Dr. Jake, one of the chief residents, to throw open the doors, get the laboring women lined up for the OR. We hear the women moaning or screaming or, the good ones, just making quiet little cries, split like squabs before the knife. And Dr. Brown stands, right there in the hall, spreads their naked legs and shoves his hand up to check the dilation, without even a greeting or an attempt to shield. It's hard for us, callous as we are, let alone the young students, to see.

We, ourselves, are not without feeling, though our lives are beyond the imagining of these doctors. We're women, too, we've known that moment the baby comes, the sudden spitting out of life. We don't doubt Dr. Brown's skill and value, but we know how embarrassing childbirth is, and how your pride just has to bend aside. When it's over, though, you've got your baby to grab onto, and what joy could be more clear?

"I have requested this meeting to make something perfectly clear," says Dr. Brown, flexing his jaw, and running his hand over his bald spot.

"Lord," whispers the Five South aide to the RN, "I called housekeeping twice about that sink," she shakes her head.

"All I want to hear is that it's fixed. I've got an eclampsia and a broken monitor in room seven. And no time for this," the RN whispers back, glaring at Brown. We knew there'd be trouble with the girl, MacKenzie, and him, and here it is, already.

Dr. Brown stands at the head of the conference room table. Next to him is the nursing supervisor. If she ever does a bit of work, we'd be surprised. Brown's heavy, but sharp-creased pants and fine leather loafers show under his white coat. Our supervisor is another story entirely: the woman must study how to look like a truck, and she's just about as subtle, too. She nods and frowns at Dr. Brown's words. They both stare at the medical students and house staff who hunch up against the far wall, checking their work sheets and their watches. The two chief residents, Dr. Jake Roth and Dr. Chip, Brown's only son, sit by themselves. He's a handsome one, Chip, well built, taller than his father, and without those jowls. We see him glance at the lib girl. But once Brown starts, Dr. Chip pays close attention.

"Someone," says Dr. Brown, "has been distributing leaflets to the patients, something about so-called Patients' Rights. And Women's Rights." He stares accusingly at the assembled, who avoid his eyes. "A hospital is like a ship," he says. "There is one captain to a department, and I am that captain. I will have no one upsetting my nurses and my patients with this rot. To learn medicine is a privilege, and one which can be revoked. It is a great ignorance to think the senior doctors do not care for the patients' best interest in ways you cannot possibly yet understand.

"I know this is the current fad, all this rights business, the rights of women, of patients, of brown-haired people, let me tell you, the right that matters is the right to have your baby delivered alive and healthy. I have nothing but contempt for the kind of chairman who would allow a disruption of his wards to threaten the health and safety of mothers and children.

"No one values rights more than I. You who know my history will understand that, but we must remember that those who disrupt the efficient functioning of a maternity ward and endanger the patients in the name of so-called 'rights' are not humanists at all, but rather immature and self-centered.

"The right of mother and child to health is the principle on which I have run this department. This is what I want to make clear: whoever is found to be handing out this garbage instead of pursuing their legitimate purposes on the wards, will be sent to the Dean to be expelled or fired, whichever is the relevant punishment."

After a moment, the nursing supervisor clears her throat and says, "On behalf of the administration, I fully agree."

Having a baby seems nothing to remark on when you're young. Only when you're gray-haired can you see the Lord's hand. And, when all is said and done, what chore is more humble than to raise a child? Rules are what they need—nothing worthwhile gets made without rules. Carpenters, cooks, tailors wouldn't think to start without a plan and a measure. Just so, our own household rules. If you plant a seed in the spring, water, fertilize, weed it all summer, then come fall, you've got something to harvest. That's the way you pull up a child. We've no sympathy for rule-breakers, protesters, liberationists, whatever they call themselves; ideas make a poor substitute for hard work and common sense.

Now we see Dr. Jake pushing the lib girl down the pea-green halls to Dr. Brown. Not the brightest bulb, Dr. Jake, but well meaning and good-natured, too. It's hard on anyone to be always compared to the boss's son. There are some that think two chief residents aren't a good idea, but not us. We prefer sharing of the lead. Two horses pull a straighter plow.

"What's this about, Dr. Roth?" says Dr. Brown, looking up from the nurses' station. He's standing, a diligent leader, charts spread, making notes with which to praise and criticize his staff. He never calls residents by their first names in front of students or nurses. We like that, a touch of respect, just like Dr. Jake and Dr. Chip tell us the other way round, what with us mostly old enough to be their mothers.

"I was hustling through sign-out rounds," says Dr. Jake, holding MacKenzie by the arm, "to get to Donnelly's for a beer. You were so pissed off, I figured I'd keep my head down! But there she was, doing it smack in front of me—what could I do? So she's yours, and I'm off."

"Let me understand," says Dr. Brown, "you found Miss MacKenzie handing out those pamphlets?"

"Oh, worse than that, sir, she was sitting on their beds and reading it to them like a bedtime story, telling one of them she could refuse a C-section if she wanted! Very unprofessional, if you ask me. First thing I learned in medical school, even if it was in Mexico, never, ever, sit on the patient's bed."

"Give me that, Jake," says Dr. Brown, holding his hand out for the mimeographed, folded sheet. He looks at it for a moment then calls across to his secretary, who, like everyone else, is pretending not to listen, "Hannah, get that other one, Miss Peltier, for me."

He looks back at the leaflet and reads, "You have rights as patients and as women! You have the right to ask questions! You have the right to know who your doctors and nurses are, by name! You have the right to refuse treatment! You have the right to keep your clothes on! You have the right to privacy! Remember: childbirth is a natural act, not a sickness!"

"Did you spread this manure around my wards, Miss MacKenzie?" He looks at Mackie, the fury seeping through his face like a burn.

"I informed the women of their rights, yes," says Mackie. "I don't deny it. I told that patient she *could* refuse a Caesarian, not she *should.* I told her you should be helping her understand."

"You tell them they have a choice," barks Dr. Brown, "the poor girls will say 'No,' and kill their babies. I can promise you, it will happen."

"Excuse me, Dr. Brown," says Jake, "she was only explaining things to them, nicely, too."

"Shut up," says Dr. Brown. "She's toying with their lives to suit herself."

"I'm sure you're right, sir," says Dr. Jake and, running his hands through his thick curly hair, he hurries down the hall. We feel for him, caught in this storm. We feel for ourselves, too.

"On the other hand, maybe she's the one who's right," Dr. Jake says to us, and we pretend not to hear. "I'm going to get Chip," he says, and we don't answer. Jobs don't grow on trees.

"Tell me, Miss MacKenzie, what part of my order did you find unclear?" says Dr. Brown, turning back to her with a cold smile.

"It's justice," says Mackie.

"It is justice to interfere with saving life?"

"Whose life? What is saving? Brutalizing the woman's body and spirit in the process?" says Mackie, looking at him steadily. "Do you think that law, religion, philosophy, never mind the patient herself, might have anything to offer over one man's opinion?"

"You are insolent," says Dr. Brown, "and ignorant. Lots of big words won't comfort a mother with a stillborn child." He squeezes his large fingers around the leaflet, crushing it. "Should that woman refuse a Caesarian and lose her baby, I hold you directly responsible."

"You have, perhaps, confused yourself with God."

Brown starts toward Mackie, but catches himself. "You," he shouts, "have, perhaps, confused yourself with someone who might ever be a decent doctor."

"Dr. Brown," says Lucille, rushing up the hall. "Your secretary paged me?"

Brown shoves the paper at her. "Did you help her?" he says.

Lucille stops still and stares. She takes the pamphlet and reads it. "Yes," she says after a minute, "I did."

"This is my battle, Lucille," says Mackie, "you've made your choice."

"I was wrong."

"Do you think it will make it less bad for me to be expelled if you are, too?

What about your precious husband and daughter? Stay out of this, Lucille."
Mackie crosses her arms and looks away.

Lucille puts her hand on her forehead and closes her eyes. "Jesus," she says,
and groans.

"Crucifixion, as I recall," says Mackie, "necessarily precedes resurrection.
Of course, that's your religion, not mine."

"Look at them," says Brown, stepping back, "what a pair. One's a fanatic,
the other's a fool." He pauses and looks them up and down, "You're gone,
ladies, I'll toss you out myself."

Lucille sighs. "Your own son's girlfriend, best student in the class, you'd
expel her with all those loans?" she asks, looking at Mackie. "She's an orphan,
you know, since thirteen. Chip's serious, about her, I think."

"Lucille!" shouts Mackie. "That has nothing to do with it."

"Everything has to do with everything else. They always like to split things
up to suit themselves."

"There are plenty of other fish in the sea," says Brown to Lucille, waving his
hand. "Good riddance for him, if his judgment is so poor that he picks this
little barracuda. Go to the Dean's office, now. I give you seven minutes to get
across campus."

It's a lucky one who's never been crushed by life. Children are your joy and
your weakness, once you have them. Why else would we be emptying bedpans here in the stinking heat of the Bronx, while our backs grow bent and
our hair gray? Young fools, we thought we'd be different than our parents. Job
said it best: Naked came I out of my mother's womb, and naked shall I return.
That wraps it up with a ribbon and a bow.

"Dad," says Dr. Chip. We like his calmness and measure. Here's a boy who
respects the father. "Can I speak to you for a minute?"

"Are you coming to plead her case, Chip? I'll do you a favor and make it
short: no." Brown looks tired. He turns from his son but looks sideways to see
how he responds.

"You're the Chairman, Dad, it's not my position to question. I've always
admired the way you run your department. That's why I chose to train here,"
says Dr. Chip.

"You'll be happier without her, anyway," says Brown, turning back to Chip.
"A girl like that wants to turn you into her slave. Regardless, I gave a direct
order. I had to follow up. That's how you keep a department on track. Very
simple. No exceptions." He moves as if to leave.

"Dad," says Chip, "Maybe there's another way to look at it. Miss MacKenzie was just trying to do some good, and what if it was poorly thought out? She doesn't deserve to be expelled. All the years of study it took to get to medical school—one little well-intentioned slip doesn't seem to warrant such a reaction."

"Are you trying to teach me how to do my job? What do you think you know about life? My God, your mother still does your laundry," says Dr. Brown.

"People respect a man who can change his mind, Dad. They'll do more for love than fear."

"So we're talking about *love* now? That stupid girl with the child was right. She's already got you twisted around her little finger," says Brown. "Come on, Chip, think about your career."

"If you suspend Miss MacKenzie, it might have consequences you don't intend," says Dr. Chip.

"Are you threatening me, boy?"

"Take it however you want," says Dr. Chip.

"Good. I'm picking up the phone now to call the Dean. You can hear it with your own ears. I'm recommending expulsion."

"This is how you always treat women," shouts Dr. Chip. "The things you do to Mom, putting her down when she's just as smart, smarter than you, hitting on the nurses behind her back," he turns on his heel. "You're my father, but you're sick. You give me the creeps."

"Get the Dean for me, Hannah," says Dr. Brown, loudly. "Let Chip listen."

"Dr. Brown," whispers Hannah, holding her hand over the receiver, "you're recommending expelling them both?"

Dr. Brown shrugs and says, "I'm not an unreasonable man. I won't punish the other one. She, at least in the beginning, had the sense to say 'No.'"

Our mothers warned us about the heart-robbery of young men: they never think about anyone else, they flit from girl to girl, they consider the world owes them supporting, and believe me, some dumb girl's going to do it for them. But it would be wrong to say we didn't understand Dr. Chip.

We heard the girl's laughter rush down the linoleum halls, and we saw Dr. Chip stand closer to Miss MacKenzie than need be, to let himself be teased. We remembered boys when we were young, their sweetness and their heat. Even the thought softened our chores and lightened our day. Love's due a powerful respect: it's love that puts Dr. Brown and the whole ward in business. It's love that calls to life, and it's love that answers with a child.

When the Dean's office calls an hour later to say that the girl never came in, we see Dr. Brown stalk down the hall. We've grown used to MacKenzie. She's a pain, but a harder worker than most, and not too good for the lifting and the bedpans. Everyone knows she's in Post-Partum, sitting on the beds, visiting and explaining those pamphlets to the women. We try to warn her, but she just shrugs.

"I'm already expelled," she says. "It's a formality now. Let me be of use while I can." But we think we see her eyes fill. We think of our own daughters. Accommodation should be made, such high ideals, such fine goals. Why else do we yank them up into the world?

"Miss MacKenzie," roars Dr. Brown. "You are to get off my wards, out of this hospital. You have no right to be here."

"God-given right, Dr. Brown? Civil right? Moral right?" She folds her hands in her lap and looks defiantly at Dr. Brown.

"Legal right," yells Dr. Brown. "I'm calling Security."

One of the older mothers stirs from her bed down the row and says, "It's not a good thing, Dr. Brown, for you to be using force on the young girl. She's caused no harm, she's explaining to the new mums why they need come back for their check-ups, right on time."

"Mrs. Morin, isn't it?" says Brown. "Wouldn't the IRS love to have your name and date of birth?"

"Oh," says Five South Days, who's marched down the ward, followed by the aide, "that's unkind, and it's true Miss MacKenzie was causing no harm."

It's a risk for us to stand up to Brown but Evenings is hurrying up from the solarium, now, not even in uniform yet. The ward secretaries stand in the door.

He turns to us, throws up his arms, and says, "No harm? Refusing a Caesarian when you need one is not harm?" He paces up and down a minute, tightens his jaw, then says, "You think she defends the patients? No, she sets herself apart."

"What are you accusing me of now?" says Mackie, narrowing her eyes and rising.

"You would have these women," Dr. Brown gestures to the patients, "attended by doctors who've never learned what they are doing. Doesn't the Lib movement think doctors should be better trained in dealing with women's problems? How are they supposed to learn if not on patients?"

"You can ask for consent, treat the women with respect. Take a little of your time and effort to explain," Mackie tilts her chin and stares at Dr. Brown.

"Ah, the worm turns. And you think that in the middle of labor or some other difficulty they can really consent? You don't think they would feel they had to say yes? What uneducated woman can really understand the issue, especially at a time like that?" Brown pauses and smiles, "If you really felt our teaching should improve, that patients are exploited for teaching, you would give a little of your own time and effort. This is what I've heard other women do: volunteer themselves. Or are you too good for that?"

There is a silence, then Mackie says, furiously, "My goodness is not for someone like you to decide." She storms from the room.

"That is an example," yells Brown after her, "of why they call you the weaker sex."

We should have intervened, we should have disallowed it. She's a proud one with her head in the clouds, never thinking her body might be attached. Dr. Brown senses the weakness like a wolf on a kill. He taunts and confuses her with his logic. Not us.

It's a hard thing to be young and female and have an opinion. Look at that movie about Joan of Arc. She ended up on the stake, but what man would have tolerated her power? It was death for her, one way or another. Look at Tina Turner. Look at that head nurse from surgery, got a raise the week after her ex was fired, so he shoots her. We tell our daughters, don't wear short skirts, don't speak out of turn, don't walk alone at night, don't catch their eye. If you must be a hero, wait until you're older and they won't get so worked up.

Dr. Brown looks at the Dean and sees a man bent with time, thick glasses falling down his nose. But still, when he summons, Brown must come.

"I wanted to talk to you, Sandy, I've heard a little about what's happened with this girl, Louise MacKenzie. I wanted to hear it from you."

"It's quite straightforward," says Brown, leaning back in the overstuffed couch and putting his arm across its broad back. "The girl was insolent and insubordinate. She disrupted the teaching ward. I made it clear she would be expelled if she did not stop, and she did not. That's all there is to it."

"The power to expel lies only with the Dean's office," says the Dean. "It's a severe punishment. I worry that you've made a mistake."

"If you don't agree, find some other way for her to learn OB/GYN. It's nothing to me," says Brown. He examines the window with its slatted shade tipped against the sun.

"No, Sandy, listen. You've gotten that department in the best shape it's ever been. This is truly admirable. But I've heard distressing things lately. Your junior faculty is unhappy; your son, a fine young man, is against you. This girl, MacKenzie, there's a lot of sympathy. I've even heard from nurses. Take care, old friend," the Dean points a wavering finger, "the other hospitals all would like to have the overall Chair. Your position isn't secure."

"You think that allowing chaos on the wards is the way to keep my position? We have a difference in administrative style." Brown smiles, resting his head back and half-closing his eyes, still watching the Dean.

"Think back, Sandy, to your own youth. Weren't you idealistic and absolute? Sandy, we all know your heroism at that age," the Dean sits forward. "The young are often not wrong, Sandy, just immoderate."

"She's not fighting a war. I put my life, my body on the line for my ideals. You know I objected to admitting girls and this is why: women will never have the judgment and courage of men, they'll never be asked to fight or give their lives, they just don't have the mind or strength for it. And who knows better than I their weaknesses, their pregnancies, their hormonal dependence. Let them be nurses, teachers, whatever. Just keep them out of my department."

The Dean shakes his head. "I won't expel her, Sandy. And if you had any sense of self-preservation, you'd make her repeat the course, but let her back in. Give a little, Sandy. Or your whole department may shatter. Your family, too." He rises from behind his desk and reaches out to shake Brown's hand. Brown rises, too.

"She insults me, she interferes with my wards, she endangered a patient, she flirts with my son, and she dresses like a whore," he says. "If she stays it's on my terms or not at all," and he bares his teeth in a smile before he leaves.

We're tired of trouble and try not to see Dr. Jake rushing, sweating and red-faced up to Brown's office, but we see him anyway and we're worried. Dr. Brown's wife is there, a former nurse herself, concerned about her husband and her son. We're more inclined to action than prayer, but we find a moment, now: let us be a vessel for healing, let tomorrow come no worse than today. A hospital can rightly aim no higher. Thy will, not mine; we know our place.

Jake runs to Dr. Brown's secretary. "Oh it's terrible, Hannah," he says, "terrible. I don't know what to do. He teased her a little, but so what?"

"Jake," says Hannah, glancing at the open door to the office. Mrs. Brown is standing inside, just hidden from view; she's come answering Hannah's call. Hannah motions Jake to lower his voice, but he doesn't understand.

"She worked herself up to it, Hannah, organized it, told them all to come to clinic, even though she's supposed to be gone. The girl, MacKenzie, she'd decided she should teach on herself, can you imagine that? I thought Dr. Brown would say enough's enough, but when he finds out he grabs me and we hurry right down to Outpatient, the nurses are fit to be tied. They'd called the supervisor, but she's in a meeting."

"Jake," says Hannah.

"Yeah, so, anyway, she's in there, looking a little pale, the guys all in a circle around the examining table. She's prepped like a patient, naked, you know, down below. It takes me a minute to grasp and Dr. Brown stops, but Mackie ignores him and keeps lecturing. I guess that does it, because he yanks on a glove, says, "I admire your dedication, young woman," and goes right to her most private places. She looks startled, closes her knees for a moment, but he pushes them back apart.

"Oh my God," says Hannah.

"'Here,' he says, spreading her, 'are the labia majora. Here the minora, here the clitoris.' The students, unsure at first, move in closer. 'A useful little organ, isn't it Miss MacKenzie? Or should I ask my son?'"

"Quiet, Jake," says Hannah, covering her eyes.

"And Mackie's face gets even whiter," Jake goes on. " 'At least as useful as a penis,' she says, but her voice is shaking."

"'Usually,' he says, 'the speculum should be warmed,' and he shoves it into her, just like that. She cries out."

Hannah moans, but she keeps listening now, hooked like a fish on a line.

"Just then, the door flies open and it's Chip, all unshaven from being on-call. Chip and Lucille, the two she wouldn't tell. They woke Chip up, Lucille's right on his heels."

"Dr. Brown doesn't even turn. 'But I've been told it is dehumanizing,' says Brown, 'to show the woman as just a part, that it is better to have no sheet at all,' and with his left hand, he whips off the sheet so that Mackie lies there, entirely naked like a little white sacrifice, skewered before our eyes."

"Stop," says Hannah to Jake. She stands up to grab him, but he steps away, consumed by his story, his eyes fixed on hers, needing to tell. She sits back down and buries her head in her arms. "Quiet," she says, "Rose is in there," but Jake doesn't even pause.

"'No!' Chip shouts at his father. 'You bastard.' He stands right in front of Dr. Brown and hits him, *pow,* on the chin, sends him back against the wall. Now the students . . . and I must admit, I myself, have no idea what to do. 'Hey,' says one of them, trying to hold Chip back."

"'Chipster,' I say. Lucille is releasing the speculum, grabbing the sheet off the floor and wrapping it around Mackie."

"'You should have let me, Mackie,' she says. 'If it had to be done, oh Mackie, it would've been easier for me.' She holds her tight, and Mackie sits up, straight and trembling, but proud."

"Chip breaks away from us and throws his father back against the wall, hard. Dr. Brown's no match for him, you know, Chip's taller, and he boxed in college. He's letting loose, now."

"'You're fired,' " says Dr. Brown with his mouth bleeding, and his nose, too."

"Oh, no," moans Hannah.

"'You're revolting,' says Chip. 'Shall I teach a rectal on you? Maybe a genital exam?'"

"'Chipster,' I try again."

"'Shut up!' he screams. 'You think he's a great doctor? He's just a dirty old man. He's screwed every nurse he could in this hospital and the secretaries, too.'"

"Stop!" shouts Hannah. "Stop it now."

"No, listen Hannah, Chip goes on, 'And I have to lie about it to Mom, not any more! God, he makes me sick. Fired, fine. I quit. I quit chief resident, I quit medicine, I quit son. I have no father. No wonder he doesn't have relatives. He doesn't deserve them.'"

Hannah has put her hands to her ears, but Jake keeps going.

"We're all watching Dr. Brown now, and I must say, he does look sick. No more yelling out of him, he's just wiping his face on his coat and watching Chip. Chip turns to Mackie and reaches out."

"'If you think you did this for me, Chip,' she says, her jaw clenched even though she's crying, 'you're mistaken. This was between you and your father, and I had nothing to do with it.'"

"Chip stares at her like she'd hit him. After a minute he leaves, just like that. Then I leave, too, thinking I'd better get back and call for help, not that I've any idea who can help. Let me sit down here, and you figure it out. Dr. Brown needs a surgeon. Miss MacKenzie needs someone, too. And Chip, I'm afraid for him. Who knows what he'll do?"

Dr. Jake sits down and we sit, too, overcome. Even with a busy ward, some things require thought. Before we can really reflect, a slender, gray-haired woman runs out of the office, head down, scurrying, almost, except it's done with a sort of grace.

"Mrs. Brown, Rose," calls Hannah, "he didn't mean it," but Mrs. Brown has rounded the emergency exit, and now it shuts with a metallic bang.

"Jake," says Hannah, "what are we going to do?"

And we must say, all women as we are, that we know what Mrs. Brown's going to do: divorce him. To a wife, the husband is rarely worth more than the son. Dr. Brown misjudged that one by a mile. We're sorry for the girl, Mackie, too, but a woman's a fool to think she has the freedoms of a man. Dr. Brown's wife knows better. She'll go with her son, do his laundry, and we would, too. There's more comfort being poor with appreciation than well-off treated like a slave.

Room five is calling for pain meds, room seven isn't progressing, and there are twins down in the emergency room. All this excitement hasn't stopped the work, nor will it, and we hope Dr. Brown comes back soon. He's a good obstetrician, we'd trust our lives to him, and who would know better than us? No one's perfect, great men have great faults. Brown will be our chairman regardless of wife and son, or how he treats female medical students. And we'll respect his work. That's our first business, the health of mother and child. That and earning a living, that's what counts for us.

And so the wards go on, women labor, babies arrive, and, two weeks later, Dr. Brown returns. He goes back to work as if nothing had happened, just he's a little quieter now, and that's okay; how could his punishment be any more clear? He lost everything: wife, child, power. The girl, of course, lost more. But life stops for no one, even though we wish it would. The Lord gives and the Lord takes away. When you and I pass from dust to dust, the sun will rise and there'll still be work to be done the next day.

Twenty-five years later, our daughters watch Dr. Lucille Peltier read a formal-looking note tacked on the board outside her office: "We are saddened to inform the Medical School community that Dr. Sandy Brown, dedicated and superb teacher of generations of students, passed on last month. There are no survivors." Lucille takes a deep breath, the hallway smells of cleansers.

She walks into her office and looks around, at the glossy black chair with the medical school emblem on its curved back, at the bookcase filled with texts, at the carpet, attractive but tweedy, to cover the dirt. She looks at the Teacher of the Year Certificates on her wall, six of them, and a Certificate of Appreciation from the Women Medical Students' Association, too. Her spare fingers pick up a framed photo from her desk. It is the picture of her daughter, a tall, smiling girl, dressed in cap and gown, waving a diploma in the air, triumphantly.

Lucille sits down behind her desk and pulls, one more time, the postcard from behind the photo. It is curled and frayed, but legible:

Dear Lucille, you were so kind to write. The Dean suggested a leave so I'm staying with my cousin for a while. Of course it wasn't a rape—I chose it myself. We have to be careful to not overuse that word. Besides, I think that I was wrong. I'm sorry to hear about your divorce. It didn't work out with Chip and me, either, though, or maybe because he cut off his father entirely, including quitting medicine and changing his name! Give my best to your little girl, it's hard for me to go back after everything that happened, but I'm just going to make myself. See you soon, love, Mackie

Lucille leans back and stares at Dr. Brown's Psalm. *The Lord is my Shepherd.* She remembers kneeling, church splintered, in her lacy white dress. *I shall not want.* She has a department strong in primary care, lowest maternal and infant mortality in the city. Inherited from him.

"Hannah," she says to her secretary, who is scheduled to retire soon, "I heard Louise MacKenzie's out of work. I'm going to offer her that job."

"The slot's for family medicine," says Hannah, while she reaches for the phone. "She's an internist, and she hasn't had an academic job in years. Isn't she divorced now, with two kids?" But she's already checked the directory and she's dialing. "How're you going to get that past the committee?"

"Those only appear to be the rules," says Lucille. "The real rules are different."

"What do you mean, you're a failure," Lucille shouts at Mackie, a minute later. "Your daughter, Mackie, your son. Set an example." She lowers her voice, "I'll walk in the building with you if that will help." She listens. "Please, Mackie, you were first in the class. Don't let them win," she says, "please."

As for us, we're old now. We sit in our beds, lean on our canes, watch television with earphones in the parlor. We're quiet after a lifetime of birth. We find our tongues bathed and wrapped with song. We don't know if wisdom comes with age, but we do know this: shave, prep, enema, scrub, we cup our hands to the river of birth that runs crowning over. Yes, indeed, we've done our job. And surely now, goodness and mercy shall follow.

Call

David Hellerstein

It's like a dream, coming into the city at this hour, no traffic on the Brunckner, the FDR Drive practically empty except for the odd security guard coming off shift and a caravan of befuddled Nebraska tourists waggling across the middle lane, and I even get a spot right in front of the hospital, where ambulettes are usually double-parked, idling at midday. I am actually early, so I drop into my office for a moment to check my e-mail, then swing up to the inpatient service, where three of the four docs sit in the residents' office. The fourth is nowhere to be found.

"Let me beep him," says Jan Virkowski, a sardonic Romanian who is the senior resident On Call tonight. Somehow he has come up with a tuna fish sandwich for breakfast, which rests on the grimy desk in front of him.

The room stinks. It is a typical residents' office: coffee-stained carpeting, smeared windows that will not open, unruly piles of lab printouts and drug company promotional materials. This is where they see their patients during their inpatient rotation.

Virkowski punches numbers into the phone, and we wait. I am Attending On Call this weekend, and there is one senior resident beside Virkowski, namely Sula Patria, an Indian woman; and one junior, Petrucelli, a lanky young Californian with a tattoo on her right shoulder, and four earrings in one ear.

"Sorry, sorry that I am late," says Ross. "I went down by the ER on my way here, it was a mistake." He rushes into the room, his white coat crisp and fresh, so freshly shaven that his jaw resembles blue stone. "So, how does it look?"

"Beds everywhere," says Virkowski.

Ross groans.

"Okay, let's get started," says Petrucelli. "We have four admissions from Friday night."

Before she can begin, though, Dr. Patria interrupts. "I don't usually tell about consults," she says. "But this one may be a problem."

Mrs. Drummond, as I will call her, is a fifty-two-year-old widow, admitted to the medicine service by her internist. Five weeks ago, for reasons known only to Mrs. Drummond, she entirely stopped eating. Her weight is down to 80 percent of normal.

"She needed intravenous hydration," Patria said, "and once her pressure was back up, her daughter wanted to sign her out. The floor called me last night at 10:00 P.M.—they want to discharge her today."

"And what's the problem?"

"She's going to die. If she keeps starving herself, she won't last more than a few weeks. But, the problem is, her internist wants to let her go. I think he's in denial about the seriousness of the problem."

"You want to transfer her to Psychiatry?"

"She won't sign in!"

"And she's not 2Pc-able?" That is, admissible against her will.

Patria shakes her head. "Only if she was at 75 percent normal body weight."

This is why I'm here. I am Attending On Call this weekend, the second of two weeks in this cycle. Twice a year, each of us attending psychiatrists carries the On Call beeper for our department. It didn't used to mean much—it was more of a conversation starter than anything.

"Gee, why do you have *two* beepers?" some parent would ask when you stood on the sidelines at your kid's soccer game.

"Oh, I'm on call for the hospital," you would say. "And for my practice."

There was a vague macho feeling involved, like carrying two six-shooters. But really, you never did anything. The residents never called you—out of respect for your sleep time, perhaps, or out of their own macho pride. This thing being, when Monday came around, major problems could have festered undetected for days. So the Chairman clamped down. Now we have to go in on weekends, and Round with the Residents. We have to see every new admission, examine them, write a note. Generally, we just give our blessing to what the residents have decided. And do our best that nothing will go wrong on our shift.

Never mind the lecture hall and anatomy dissections and morning Rounds—every young medical student and resident knows how important Call is. Nights and weekends are when all the real action happens in hospitals, when decisions have to be made and lives saved. Call is where students become doctors.

In my own life, Call began at an early age, long before I entered medical school. When I was a kid, my dad, a cardiologist, in his months of "on service," would often need to go down to the hospital to help the residents. And not infrequently, he would bring me with him. It was a central part of my childhood, driving down the hill to University Hospital late at night, parking in the Doctors' lot, and going up to the medical floors to see a patient who was doing badly, whom the residents and fellows On Call couldn't stabilize. Wearing an oversized, borrowed white coat, which dragged on the floor behind me, I would follow Dad along long gleaming corridors to the Coronary Care Unit.

There, the white-coated doctors would crowd intently around Dad, reporting their problems and dilemmas. I would watch them all, lit by the green oscilloscopes, as Dad flipped through the chart, unrolling long waxy EKG tapes, as he began to decode the mysteries that were baffling them. Doctoring seemed incredibly exciting then, incredibly glamorous, almost holy.

After what seemed like an indeterminable delay, Dad would say, "Let's go see the patient," and the troops would gather together and follow him away. Generally I would be left at the nurses' station, but as I got older, increasingly, I would be asked along too, and, feeling like an imposter, would join the white-coated crowd up at the bedside where some blue-faced elderly gentleman was propped up, gasping for air.

A decade or so later, as a medical student and a young doctor-in-training, taking Call became positively exciting. Being on the frontlines, one had the feeling of trench warfare. There were always new admissions, bleeding or arresting or seizing or groaning in pain. There was always something to do STAT. One day, on surgery rotation in my third year of med school, there arrived a postman who, in a bizarre attempt to kill himself, had taken a box cutter and sliced a hundred times across his body—all the way down to muscle. The surgery resident and I spent an entire afternoon suturing him. It was incredible—to be able to perfect my technique while at the same time saving the guy's life!

That was only one adventure On Call. There was always something, and even in the moments of tedium, there was the hospital as a set, a twenty-four-hour theatre throbbing with possibilities. The internal hospital hallways, the soggy sandwiches grabbed from vending machines and the unending supply of 2:00 A.M. pizzas, the beepers that wouldn't stop squawking, the central line trays and the chest tube setups wrapped as carefully in their blue cloth as holy scrolls. Such is the stuff of every doctor's private legend.

But these days my life is less glamorous, both during the workday and when I am taking Call. Days, I spend much of my time, as do thousands of hospital doctors, training young doctors, reviewing their cases, making sure their documentation is up to par. I have become part of "administration." What are we hospitals "administering"? I know my residents might answer that question. But at the risk of pretentiousness, I would say that we are administering care. Though far less thrilling than the life-and-death dramas that present every day in the emergency room, our work is nonetheless important in saving lives—just like clean drinking water prevents many more deaths than high-tech heart operations.

And when we Attendings are taking Call—well, sometimes it is like being at Mission Control, watching one's astronauts ascend into space. Like grounded space-travelers, we watch our students rocketing above, full of wistful pride as they leave vapor trails behind them, disappearing into blackness. Other times, we feel like glorified driving instructors, sitting beside our novice drivers as we barrel unsteadily down the highway, resisting most impulses to grab the wheel.

Despite the loss of glamour, I reassure myself: *It is okay. It is necessary and good.* After all, one cannot be a student forever. And this is where so much healing occurs—in quiet conversations between doctors in hospital wards, in reports and summaries and bedside examinations.

But something is different today. Last weekend, the beginning of my On Call cycle, seems like a hundred years ago. In the interim has come an announcement of our hospital's immense financial crisis.

"A forty-, maybe fifty-million-dollar deficit this year," our Chairman announced this past Monday in our Executive Committee meeting. "Maybe one hundred million next year. Things aren't likely to improve in the foreseeable future."

We—the senior Attending docs—sat in stunned silence. Ten or twenty million in deficit would not have surprised us. But fifty million is immense.

Within a day or two, rumors became rampant. It doesn't help that, as *Crain's Business Weekly* has reported, Moody's downgraded the hospital system's bonds to junk. Things are so bad, we hear, that the hospital president's limo driver has been laid off. And Pediatrics—Pediatrics!—may be shut down! At our sister hospital, part of the same hospital system, Dentistry has abruptly been closed. "And it wasn't even losing money!" they say.

In Psychiatry, my Outpatient division is going to bear the brunt of the cuts. It is not a matter of trimming or scrimping—which we have done innumerable times before. We will have to close something, most likely our Day Treatment Program. Most of its staff will be let go. Perhaps we can squeeze an MD into my clinic, and a few social workers into vacancies on Inpatient, but the nurse and other staff will be fired. One woman comes into my office in tears. Just married, and pregnant, her husband unemployed, she does not know what she will do. Disconsolate, she just sits there, as if waiting long enough will bring her job back.

Even on the inpatient service, morale is low. Just two days ago, a psychotic girl was attacked by a street-wise addict, also a patient, in the middle of the day. No staff was around in time to intervene.

And so, within a week, our normally bustling hospital has taken on a sense of siege. In the hallways, the doctors who are always standing before elevator banks quietly consulting about their patients, or rushing through the park on the way to their floors, are now silent with worry, pale with rage. What is happening to our beloved hospital, which has been serving the Lower East Side for over 100 years? How can we be abandoning our patients?

Thus it is almost a relief to go On Call again, to see the circumscribed misery of each new admission, and to know that we can help, at least for this "episode of illness."

After the case presentation, we go on Walk Rounds to see them. There is a seventeen-year-old girl who took an OD of ibuprofen after her boyfriend left her. A Central Park West mother who convinced the ER attending that she needed a break from her desperate life that only the inpatient psychiatric unit could provide. And a Latino man with gangbanger tattoos, who can't help grinning when he tells us how "depressed" he is. Why is he trying to con us? Who knows, maybe he needs to get off the streets for a few days.

And then there is Mr. Tagore, an admission from last weekend who is still here. His father brought him to the U.S. two years ago. In Pakistan he had been in one mental hospital after another, receiving terrible treatment. Once he got to the U.S., he stayed in a single-room-occupancy hotel, getting worse and worse, until the old man finally brought him into the hospital. Last weekend, on our Rounds, he was locked behind a door with a small reinforced-glass window. Crouched down on the floor, naked, he was eating out of a plastic cereal bowl with his fingers. He'd been drinking his own urine, the nurse told us. So we had increased his antipsychotic right away.

Today, though, Mr. Tagore is incredibly improved. Now dressed in crisply pressed hospital pajamas, he walks around the unit arm-in-arm with his attendant, a Filipino woman. He nods to us, wordlessly smiling in gratitude.

What about the starving woman? The convention is that we don't round on the consultations from the medical floors. I know Virkowski would see it as a rebuke if we were to break protocol and do so, so I never see the patient I am most worried about.

Instead, Virkowski and I strategize about how he should handle her case: what if she insists on signing out today?

And that is it. After I have interviewed each patient briefly, we stand in the nurses' station conversing. Then the residents rush off to order labs, write their notes, and see what's happening in the ER. I write my notes, and then it is time for me to go home.

I had worried that Virkowski would not be as concerned about Mrs. Drummond as Dr. Patria had been. Perhaps it is his Slavic fatalism, his Eastern European world-weariness, I mused, or maybe he just isn't as good of a resident as Patria. Whatever the cause, as we discussed Mrs. Drummond's case, he seemed more laissez-faire, as if to say, "Let that lady do what she wants. If she wants to kill herself, who are we to stop her?" Even though, as we both agreed, she was a highly atypical case for self-starvation.

Yet scarcely an hour after I have left the hospital he is ringing me up on my cell phone, sounding scared.

"Mrs. Drummond's daughter is here. She wants to take her mother home now. What am I supposed to do?"

I am back in suburbia—in fact, in the middle of a vast Price Club warehouse, pushing a huge shopping cart piled with oversized cartons of pasta, soup, and canned fruit. The reception is not good. "Technically she has the right to leave," I say. "But I think . . . I think you should try to play for time."

"And what will that accomplish?" asks Virkowski.

"Tell her," I say, "that unless she starts eating she can't go home."

It is a modest lie, but worth trying. My guess is that even if we did transfer her to Psychiatry against her will, it would be unlikely to help unless she has some inkling of how severe her problem is.

"And if she really insists on leaving?"

I think for a moment. "I guess I would refuse to let her go unless her internist comes in to see her. Let *him* sign her out. Do you want to take responsibility for her life?"

I know that the odds of him coming in today are nil.

"No," says Virkowski, and adds reluctantly, "Okay, I will try that."

He calls again after dinner. He sounds exhausted. He tried my line, he says, that she had to eat in order to leave. They haven't been able to reach Mrs. Drummond's doctor, despite calling his service, paging him, and so on.

"The daughter, she got tired of waiting and went home. She says, okay, her mother will stay tonight, but she is insisting to take her home tomorrow. She'll call a lawyer, she will sue us if we don't let her go. Doctor," he adds plaintively, "What is the point of all this? We are only bluffing."

"When you're On Call," I say, "sometimes you have to bend the rules."

"For what end?"

I don't know how to answer that question. I am hardly optimistic. "We have to do what we can," I say finally.

The next morning, Sunday, is a variation on Saturday. Again there is no traffic on the Drive, and again I slide easily into Doctors' parking, and again there are three residents waiting for me in the grimy inpatient office. Virkowski has yet another tuna fish sandwich on the desktop before him. And again there is no sign of Ross.

"Sorry, sorry that I am late," says Ross, finally making an appearance. "I went down by the ER on my way here, it was a mistake." He rushes into the room, his white coat now crumpled and stained, his jaw covered with stubble. He carries an enormous Dunkin Donuts iced coffee, which he immediately proceeds to spill.

"So, how does it look?" asks Dr. Lewii, the junior resident who is coming on service.

"Beds everywhere! We only had two admissions."

She groans. She is a soft-faced Israeli who has just finished serving her Army term. Kiplander, the new senior resident, American born, looks about fifteen years old, so that I practically expect him to cruise down the halls on one of those shiny aluminum scooters.

Dabbing the carpet with napkins, Ross continues to talk.

"We have Mr. Shea, an Irish man from Bensonhurst, an extremely severe alcoholic, and Mrs. Berhkinskov, a pharmacist from Russia."

He rushes through the presentation of their cases, and then everyone gets up, ready to go over the floor.

"What about the other case?" I ask.

"Nothing new," Virkowski says. He last saw her at 8:00 P.M.—nothing had changed. He describes her to Kiplander, who listens quietly, with a puppy-like air. Will this young kid be able to stand up to Mrs. Drummond's daughter? I have my doubts.

Both patients are in the other building. We walk outside.

Three fire-trucks have pulled up in front of the building entrance, and half-a-dozen firefighters holding hoses and axes stand in the lobby, having commandeered the elevators. So we go around to the First Avenue entrance, and up to the sixth floor. The only way to get to the psych ward from here is to go through Pediatrics, the unit that is being closed.

"They'll never let us go through," whispers Dr. Lewii as we approach.

The Peds nurses look up, surprised.

"There's a fire," I say. "They've cut off the elevators. Can we walk through your unit?"

They nod us through the nearly empty ward.

Over on Psychiatry, we find Mr. Shea, a ruddy-faced man with two black eyes. With merciless clarity he describes his own certain doom. "Both of my parents died of drink," he tells us. "I know how it's going for me. Already, my liver is hot. I know what I oughta do is stay clean, only I can't do it!"

Mrs. Berhkinskov is an ancient crone who it turns out is only thirty-eight years old. In broken English she explains how five of her neighbors have keys to her apartment, and enter it whenever she leaves, stealing her valuables.

"This is very unusual," I tell Dr. Lewii. "She needs to be worked up for dementia."

After rounds, I write my notes. I review Mrs. Drummond one last time with Kiplander, and then it is time for me to leave.

Outside, it is still quiet. In front of the hospital, where ambulettes are usually pulled up, idling, and where Hasids from Williamsburg are always sitting in battered Pontiacs, waiting for their bewigged wives, the street is practically empty.

A Latino family walks slowly toward me, kids and grandma and parents, dressed for church.

I am just pulling out of my parking space when I get paged. It is Kiplander, sounding excited.

"Doctor!" he cries. "I need to tell you! Mrs. Drummond's daughter is here! She wants to take her mother back home!"

His voice crackles through my cell phone. I pull back to the curb.

"You know what we talked about," I say.

"No, no, I think she can leave. Her internist has already come by. And she has an appointment to see the psychiatrist tomorrow. And guess what?"

She started eating, he tells me. Last night, after Virkowski left the floor, she had a full dinner. And this morning, breakfast as well.

I listen to him, trying to dissect the truth from his enthusiasm.

"She swears she'll keep it up!" he cries.

Naturally, I feel a need to temper his excitement. People will say anything, do anything, to get out of the hospital. But I wonder: is there perhaps some hope for Mrs. Drummond?

There is a feeling at the end of Call that is difficult to describe. Relief, of course—and fatigue, even if you have gotten a good night of sleep, since you've been carrying a heavy load of possible disaster. But there is satisfaction as well—at least when you have reason to believe that you have taken care of today's problems, and perhaps prevented a few disasters. I can remember, after Dad stabilized the patients in the Coronary Care Unit, the feeling of driving back up Cedar Hill, and when we came home in the dark, still house, where Mom and all my brothers and sisters were sleeping, and when we sat in the breakfast room, snacking on fried bologna with ketchup on rye, or boiling some hot dogs—always some kind of junk—and the feeling that we would have, or the feeling of Dad's that I would share. Something good had been done. Someone would live. I got the same feeling that day in med school when we took out the postman's last stitches, and wrote orders for antibiotics, and went out into the hospital parking lot for a breather and a Coke.

And so it is today, with Mrs. Drummond. Sure, tomorrow I have to go back to the hospital's problems, to the layoffs and the deficit and the programs that we need to close.

But with this Call, speaking for myself and the residents, it is fair to say that we have done what had to be done. And maybe we have made a little bit of a difference. In the end, as a doctor, that's the best you can hope for.

Alpha-1

Perri Klass

I WORK AT A neighborhood health center. I do pediatric primary care. I like my job, I like watching the kids grow up, and I worry about all the usual primary care bugaboos: will I pick it up early enough if a baby has congenital dysplasia of the hip—if you catch it early, it's relatively easy to fix; if you miss it, it can mean big time surgeries, months in a body cast—for an infant!—and, worst of all, permanent damage to the hip joint. Or how about, will I miss a meningitis—winter comes, and the clinic sessions are full of kids with high fevers and headaches and upper respiratory symptoms—in other words, with flu. If one of them actually has meningococcal meningitis brewing, given that the early symptoms can be high fever, headache, upper respiratory symptoms, along with stiff neck and vomiting, will I pick the kid out? Or will I wait for the later symptoms—shock, seizures, coma, death? Yes, indeed, as I said, I worry about the usual primary care everyday problems, the big ones and the little ones. Appendicitis. Walking pneumonia. Swimmer's ear. Scoliosis. Urinary tract infections. Head lice.

One thing about doing pediatric primary care in a neighborhood health center is that you don't see many rare or extreme diseases. When the medical students rotate through, they are often delighted by our health center, impressed by the camaraderie of the pediatric group, touched by our involvement with our patients and their families, respectful of all the many programs we coordinate to reach beyond the clinic and help children with their home environments, their school issues, their daily lives. But medical students rarely find their "great cases," their remarkable medical stories, their tertiary care miracles, in the crowded exam rooms and the busy hallways of the health center. You don't come to us for high-tech medicine, or for big-ticket subspecialty heroics. So of course, this is the story of my patient who needed the big-ticket, high-tech subspecialty heroics. My "great case." This is the story of Catriona.

She was born in the winter, three and a half years ago. In fact, in the best women's magazine tradition, she was a holiday season baby, born into an Irish family with two older children. She was small at birth, what we call in the trade "borderline sGA," meaning that she was almost below the cut off for being identified as an unexplainably small, full-term infant (sGA is the acronym for "Small for Gestational Age"). But she was on the right side of the borderline, so she didn't get worked up for the things you usually think about with sGA babies—congenital infections like cytomegalovirus and toxoplasmosis. She was on the right side of the borderline, so she went home at the age of two days, and came into the health center for a check a couple of days later. We weighed her on our baby scales, and I noted that she was small, but growing, clinging to the bottom of the growth curve. She was a vigorous, good-natured baby. I thought I should see her a little more frequently than we usually see newborns just because she was so small; I wanted to make sure she kept growing.

But then she came back for one of those return visits, and her mother had a question: did I think the baby looked jaundiced? Joan was an experienced mother; she knew infant jaundice was common and was worth worrying over. And in fact that's another one of the standard primary care worries—neonatal hyperbilirubinemia, the yellow/orange tinge to a baby's skin caused by the buildup of bilirubin pigments in the blood, left over from the breakdown of old red blood cells. The pigment builds up as the baby breaks down red cells because the immature newborn liver doesn't do a good job of getting rid of bilirubin. Babies are at especially high risk for hyperbilirubinemia if they are chewing up their red blood cells faster than usual for one reason or another. As a pediatrician, you have to worry about it because if the bilirubin gets way, way high, it can cross from the newborn blood into the newborn brain, because the newborn blood-brain barrier is leaking, and in the newborn brain, bilirubin can cause brain damage. This condition, called kernicterus, is fortunately rare, but fear of kernicterus keeps us checking blood bilirubin levels on a lot of babies, and sometimes hospitalizing them for phototherapy—days spent under ultraviolet lights which help break down the pigment.

So here was this little tiny relatively newborn infant whose mother thought she looked jaundiced—I immediately performed the first sophisticated health center diagnostic test—I held the baby up to the window. Lots of people look a little yellow under fluorescent lights; daylight is much more reliable. We always hold babies up to the window when we're trying to decide whether they're jaundiced. And this baby didn't look jaundiced, but her color did look a little funny to me—kind of pasty, kind of unhealthy. But definitely not yellow. And otherwise she looked fine, alert and active, and her weight was again up a little—same bottom-of-the-growth-chart line. I asked a colleague to come look at her with me, our usual next diagnostic step in assessing possible neonatal jaundice: just how yellow does this baby look to you? Yellow enough to have the family go home and come back tomorrow? Yellow enough to draw blood and check a bili level? Yellow enough to hospitalize (what we call in the trade, a pumpkin baby, or sometimes, a glow-in-the-dark pumpkin baby)? My colleague was a pediatric nurse practitioner who used to work as a neonatology nurse. She looked at Catriona and agreed with me that she wasn't very yellow. "But I don't like her skin color," she said. "I wonder if she has any red blood cells in her—she looks kind of washed out and anemic."

And so of course I immediately felt stricken: she's anemic! She has no red blood cells! And I never noticed! But I sent her to get her blood drawn and told them to call me when the results came; the baby and her mother went home, and I went across town to the hospital. My beeper went off when I was in my office at the hospital, getting ready to go to the health center Christmas party. I had worn red crystal earrings that day, thinking they would look festive, and one had fallen off; I was crawling around on the floor of my office when the beeper beeped, and for some reason I still remember, almost four years later, that I answered the page while still kneeling on the floor. It was my colleague at the health center, the nurse practitioner, calling to tell me that, no, Catriona was not in fact anemic, but there was apparently something very wrong with her liver—her LFTs (liver function tests) were elevated, and it wasn't just the routine hyperbilirubinemia of a newborn. Something was wrong. We called her mother and told her to take the baby to the emergency room of the hospital where she had been born. I spoke with the emergency room pediatricians and arranged for her to be seen by a pediatric gastroenterologist, and then I located my missing earring, and I went on to the Christmas party, where I spent the evening sitting at a table with other pediatric types, discussing possible diagnoses, most of them pretty bad, for a newborn infant with liver disease.

It took a couple of weeks for the gastroenterologists to establish a definite diagnosis for Catriona. At first they just said she had "neonatal hepatitis of unknown etiology"—in other words, that she was a newborn with something wrong with her liver, thank you very much. They suspected a possible congenital infection—which would also explain why she had been born so small, of course. But the diagnosis, when all the tests finally came back in, was not infectious. Catriona had an inherited disease, an enzyme deficiency called alpha-1-antitrypsin deficiency. And, it would turn out, as yet more tests came in, she had the most severe type possible—she didn't just have low levels of the enzyme, alpha-1-antitrypsin, but almost none at all.

Alpha-1-antitrypsin deficiency can cause severe lung disease—in fact, I was most familiar with the enzyme deficiency only as something we tested for back when I was a resident when we were working up children with mysterious lung problems. Tested for and never found, I might add; I had measured the enzyme many times during my residency, but never gotten an abnormal result. As far as I was concerned, alpha-1-antitrypsin deficiency was just one of the zebras, the long list of rare-but-possible diagnoses that medical students discuss on teaching rounds and residents include on their lists, as we say, "for completeness." A zebra is a rare disease entity—an old medical joke about the student who hears hoof beats and immediately thinks of a zebra. A zebra and a lung disease, that was alpha-1-antitrypsin deficiency, as far as I was concerned. But the deficiency can also affect the liver—sometimes a little, sometimes a lot. Catriona, from the very beginning, was severely affected. She grew very slowly. Her liver got too big. Her liver functions deteriorated. She developed ascites, a condition in which fluid accumulates in the abdomen. By the time she was six months old, she had a swollen belly, with stick-like arms and legs.

"By the time she was six months old," I wrote, as if it had been routine. The truth is, of course, that a lot was going on as Catriona grew to be six months old. She was seen regularly by the gastroenterologists. Her blood was drawn to monitor the changes in her LFTS. The issue of liver transplant was discussed, first as a distant possibility, then later on as this baby's probable best hope. Catriona was also seen regularly by her primary care pediatrician, me, at the health center. I measured her head. I gave her her well baby shots, even though she certainly wasn't a well baby. Whenever I saw her name on my schedule, I would nervously look up her disease in the index of one or another of our pediatric textbooks and read what little there was, just to prep myself for the visit. I read a couple of basic articles, which focused much more on the lung disease than on the liver disease, and I kept promising myself to do some really serious research as soon as I had a chance.

Instead, Catriona's mother Joan did the really serious research. She went on the internet and found just about everything there is to be found about alpha-1-antitrypsin deficiency. She also found the association of people with the disease, and she went to the convention. She met people whose children had lung disease, people whose children had liver disease. She met someone whose child had had a liver transplant. She brought me big folders stuffed with copies of the articles she had found or been given, and guiltily, I read through them and tried to explain what seemed like the most important information, wrapping myself somewhat forlornly in the mantle of my own professional jargon.

What I had here was a child who was completely beyond my expertise. She was and would always be the first child I ever cared for with alpha-1-antitrypsin deficiency. She would probably go on to be the only child I would ever care for with this disease, though heaven knows I will test for it in future any time I see a baby with unusual skin color, or a big liver, or maybe any time I see a baby who is small at birth.

I was not competent to juggle her medications. Heaven knows I was not competent to assess the progression of her liver disease, or even to contemplate the question of a transplant. She was in the hands of experts, as she needed to be. But I sometimes felt both superfluous and silly as I asked my routine primary care questions—well, no, she wasn't trying to roll over—her belly was too big for trying to roll over! I'm not sure I would actually have used the phrase, "rearranging the deck chairs on the Titanic," but there were moments when that seemed to me the nature of my contribution. I would ask Joan what the specialists had said at her last visit, and then I would reassure her, they're very good, it's an excellent hospital, an excellent pediatric gastroenterology team. You're in good hands.

The baby came to clinic at the age of about six months, her abdomen dramatically swollen. She was a tiny girl, nothing but belly. The pressure of the fluid in her abdomen made the veins stand out blue under her skin, which was still pale and pasty. Something had gotten much worse. I didn't know how to fix it, but I knew she needed to be somewhere where people knew more than I did. So I sent her back to the emergency room, and she ended up spending almost the entire summer in the hospital, a long and scary series of medical complications. The fluid in her abdomen was drained, reaccumulated, became infected with a dangerous kind of bacteria. Her liver was tested and was discovered to be getting worse—she was headed for the very unusual complication of infant cirrhosis.

When Catriona finally left the hospital, it was with a feeding tube surgically inserted into her gastrointestinal tract and a central intravenous line surgically inserted into her chest. She was on a complex regimen of medications and vitamins, and she received continuous all-night feedings into her G-tube. The decision had been made that she was going to need a liver transplant in order to survive, and the transplant surgeons had explained to her parents that her odds of making it through the transplant would be much higher if she could grow a little. Twenty pounds, they said, we'd like her to be twenty pounds. We think she'd have a better chance.

And then began the months of trying to get Catriona up to twenty pounds, which at the beginning seemed frankly impossible. She lost what little interest in eating she had once had, and it seemed that no matter how much liquid nutrition her mother ran into her G-tube at night, she just wouldn't grow. Much of the weight gain that I had been plotting on her growth curve during her first months of life had probably been false weight—I had been weighing the fluid slowly accumulating in her abdomen, not developing muscle and bone. She hadn't been developing any muscle and bone. It was hard to look at her, sometimes, and believe she would get to twenty pounds.

That is, it was hard for me. Of course, it wasn't my job to feed her, or to juggle her medications around, or even to console her when she cried in the middle of the night. As Catriona's primary care doctor, just what were my jobs? I plotted that growth chart, of course. Sometimes I called and spoke to one of the gastroenterologists. Faithfully, I summarized their letters in Catriona's medical record at the health center—a record that was already thicker than the records belonging to most of our adolescent or adult patients. And that was about the sum total of my contribution—that and a little cheerleading for Catriona and her mother, Joan, who were actually, in their different ways, fighting this battle. Many pediatric stories have heroic mothers, both in reality and in the accumulated song, story, and folklore of my profession. And almost every parent who contends with a seriously ill child is in some sense heroic, going one-on-one with destiny, changing diapers on the edge of the abyss, singing lullabies into the void. But when I say that Joan was heroic, I mean something beyond that. Yes, she managed G-tube and central line, medication schedule and feeding schedule, and of course her older two children as well. But beyond that, she looked at Catriona and saw a child, a growing child, a child with a growing brain, and she set herself to amuse that child and stimulate that brain. Catriona was read to, sung to, talked to. Anything that interested her was brought to where she sat, solemnly, with her pale face and her blue-gray eyes and her big belly.

When Catriona was about a year old, Joan asked me whether I thought she could make some general appeal to the staff of the health center about signing organ donor cards to carry in their wallets. Catriona was going to be listed for a liver transplant, either when she reached twenty pounds or maybe even sooner, if her liver deteriorated, and Joan, through her contacts with the transplant team and the alpha-1-antitrypsin association, had become aware of the scarcity of solid organs for transplant. At some point, maybe very soon, Catriona's life would depend on getting a liver—and there aren't enough livers to go around.

I arranged to have Joan speak at one of our health center staff meetings. There were a couple of hundred people sitting in the big room. Joan brought Catriona, of course, dressed in her bright red holiday best. She held the baby, gripped the unfamiliar microphone, and faced the crowd of strangers. I'm not here because it will get my daughter a liver, she told them—I'm here because if you sign a donor card for yourself, if you donate the organs when a close relative dies, then someone who is waiting like my little girl is waiting may have a chance. She held the baby tight. Ask your priest, she told the health center employees. I asked my priest—he said the Church has no problem with organ donation. Please, please, fill out the cards, save someone. And we passed around the cards, and people took them.

Well, it took a year and a half, but Catriona grew. She got bigger, she was listed for a transplant, and her family began carrying a beeper. And then all of a sudden, as these things happen, at the speed of fatal accidents and helicopters and emergency operations, a liver was available, and Catriona went into surgery.

She did well during the long transplant procedure, and initially her recovery went well. After a week recovering in intensive care, she moved to the ward, but then had several episodes of bleeding from esophageal varices—backed-up veins in her esophagus caused by her long-standing liver problem. So they moved her back to the ICU to watch her closely, and that same day, she had a major bleed. Esophageal varices are not at all a common problem in children—they're something you're more likely to see in adults, alcoholics, say, with years of cirrhotic liver disease behind them. So the adult gastroenterologists (that is, the gastroenterologists who usually treat adults) came in and helped control the bleeding vessels. And then there were some rocky anxious days in the PICU, her mother resolutely occupying her with puzzles and toys and art projects every waking minute. The varices bled again, and were repaired again. More anxious waiting. More puzzles, more art projects.

And then she got better. To make a very long and very medical story short, Catriona is now more than a year post-transplant, still on some immunosuppressive medication, but otherwise doing fine. She's been able to eat enough to keep on growing, and the G-tube is gone, along with the central line. Her varices are resolving. Most of all, she's gone from an ill child to a well one; she eats and runs around and plays and if you saw her now, you would note curls and mischief and non-stop activity, not pallor and a distended abdomen.

The surgeons are proud of her. The transplant team, the gastroenterologists, the pediatric ICU people, they're all proud of Catriona, and they have every reason to be. And at the health center, we're proud of her too. I try to keep her out of the waiting room, since she's immunocompromised and the waiting room is full of sick people, but now and then Joan brings her by to say hello, and I exult over her chubby arms and legs, while clinic staffers who remember Joan from her staff meeting appearance stop by to say, is that your baby, she's gotten so big!

Recently, Catriona's mother applied for her to the Make-A-Wish Foundation, hoping they would arrange for Catriona to get her heart's desire—a chance to visit Mr. Rogers. I was called by someone from the foundation who basically wanted to know, now that Catriona has had her liver transplant, can she still be considered a seriously ill, even a critically ill, child? And for a moment I wanted to tell them, no, of course not. Look at her, I wanted to say, she's not sick—she's just fine! She's plump, she's growing, she's eating, her new liver is working—she's fine! But I knew better than that—and so I was honest, more honest than I wanted to be. Yes, I said, she's still high risk. She could reject the liver. She lives in an immunocompromised state. She still has this genetic disease.

I called up Joan and said I hope they grant her wish, I hope she gets to meet Mr. Rogers. And I told them the truth, I said, that as you know, she's still at risk. But from day to day, that's not how I think about her. Not any more.

And she got her wish—the foundation flew her family to Pittsburgh on Catriona's fourth birthday. A limo picked them up and took them to the public television studios, and they toured the set—Catriona saw the place where the trolley comes out, and all the other landmarks she recognized. Mr. McFeely and Mr. Aber and Lady Aberlin introduced themselves, and finally they met Mr. Rogers himself. He shook hands with Catriona, and made a point of talking with her older brother and sister as well. Catriona showed him her scar, and he was very impressed; he asked if he could take a picture of it. Catriona was very quiet around him, but never took her eyes off him, watching him almost in awe, but then he knelt beside her and they posed for pictures together.

Maybe you think you know the moral of the story. Maybe you think the moral is that she also serves who cheerleads for the mom, that in my sensitivity and my attention to primary care issues like development, I played a pivotal role in the heroic story of saving Catriona. Or that really, without my keen primary-care-trained eye for skin color or degree of abdominal distention, this child would have had no chance at all. But none of that is true. The moral of the story, at least the moral I see right now, is this: Catriona is truly a miracle child. When she runs across the playground, years of research and millions of dollars of high-tech medicine run with her. She is alive and thriving because of the dedication of her family, who fed her and cared for her and played with her and loved her, and because of the skills and training and clinical judgment of a big team of people who knew what to do for her particular disease, and watched her closely, and made the right calls. And, of course, she is alive because someone else died, and a family decided to donate a liver. And although I did not make this miracle, I have been privileged to be allowed to touch its fringes, to breathe the air of risk and possibility and hope that medical miracles diffuse. She is the other kind of primary care story—not the story of finding what you're looking out for, not the story of applying what you know to taking care of your patients. She's the story of finding something very unusual and very bad, and of what happens next.

I bring medical students in to see Catriona, on the rare occasions that she comes to the clinic to see me. I'm especially eager to bring them in and introduce them if they seem arrogant or full of themselves—here's where I show them that there's more to primary care than sniffles and diaper rash! I tell her story, proud of my ability to describe this obscure disease, which they always feel they should have heard of, but usually can't quite place, I ask them to come look at her very impressive abdominal scars, I show them her growth chart. I try to seem a little nonchalant, as if she's just *one* of the liver transplant recipients I care for here at the health center. The adventure of primary care. But sometimes I get over myself and my pretensions, as we stand there watching Catriona jump around the exam room; she never minds showing off her belly, but she gets bored with our discussions. And once I get over my own show-off impulses, what I want to say to these students is that sometimes this profession takes you down some unbelievable roads. I want them to know what she looked like as a tiny, pasty baby, and then later when she couldn't move because her belly was too swollen. I want them to understand what a sad story this started out to be, and how remarkable is the profession that turned it into something else—and which has allowed me along for the journey.

Dennis Bruce

DAVID HILFIKER

DESPITE ITS RELATIVELY small size, the basement sanctuary of St. Aloysius Church on North Capitol Street in Washington, D.C., is hardly at capacity late this Friday morning. Perhaps sixty of us cluster toward the middle, between the two rows of massive, evenly spaced pillars running from front to back and dividing the sanctuary in thirds. Nevertheless, I am surprised by how many people have chosen to attend Bruce's funeral. About a third of us are white, all members of my own faith community who have known Bruce through our various ministries to the homeless. The remaining two-thirds are African Americans. I recognize a few as former patients of mine, who probably knew Bruce from the shelters or the streets. A group of twenty or thirty—whom I assume to be Bruce's extended family—sit together toward the front. When I entered the sanctuary, I was taken aback by how many of his family were here. He has had so little contact with his family over the years and even that seems to have been difficult and painful all around. As far as I know, he has spoken with only two of his family during this past year that he has lived with us at Joseph's House, and Claudia, a younger sister, is the only one to whom he revealed his diagnosis. But funerals are perhaps the only occasion a broken family has to express its love and affection for a wayward son.

Not surprisingly, his children have chosen not to come. They would not remember him, anyway, and likely do not want to open old wounds. His ex-wife, however, sits on the other side of the center aisle. I do not know the truth of the matter, but Bruce told me several times he had walked out on her almost twenty years ago after he had returned from a stint in prison and found her in bed with someone else. He had had no contact with her afterward, he said. He told us he did not even know how to find her, so I am initially surprised she knows of his death, but I remember that word travels fast in the black community. Several cousins and their families are in attendance, and a few of them will even speak during the time that Father Anderson gives to share memories of our lives with Bruce.

As others file past the open coffin, I look around and notice five men scattered in pews, the only people sitting outside the pillars. Two sit together, but the other three are alone, physically isolated from each other and everyone else. Dressed in the dark, baggy pants and bulky coat of the street, unshaven, each looks around restlessly, as if afraid he will be asked to leave. From their leaden, almost staggering, movements, I gather they are intoxicated. These, I suspect, are Bruce's friends from the street, here to pay last respects to one of their own.

This part of North Capitol Street had been Bruce's hangout for years before he came to Joseph's House. Prior to that, he had spent time in prison for a crime he apparently did not commit. "I did lots of things just as bad," he once said, "but I was only hangin' around that alley when those guys robbed that store and shot that guy. Not even my lawyer believed me, though." One of those convicted eventually testified on his behalf, however, and Bruce was freed, but only after nine years in federal penitentiaries had come and gone. After that he was mostly homeless, frequently living in vacant buildings on this section of North Capitol Street. His last residence before Joseph's House had been one of the many abandoned houses just up the street from the church. In the last year he had asked me several times to go down with him to see that abandoned house and visit with his former drinking buddies—Mr. George, Uncle Bud, and Mike. I'd intended to. Finally his death brings me together with his friends.

A shriek pierces my reverie. Flanked by Claudia and Jeanne (the other sister I met last week), a small, dark black woman dressed in mourning advances down the far right aisle towards the casket. Suddenly she breaks and runs forward. "Noooo . . . !" she wails. "They can't take him away from me. Why him? Why did they take him away from me?" With another shriek she pitches forward and would fall into the casket if her sisters did not restrain her. This must be Denise, Bruce's twin sister. Two larger men—both in their early twenties, dark skinned, impeccably dressed in dark suits, men whom I take to be cousins—rush up and grab her under both arms. Now she is struggling and wailing; her feet no longer support her. I am suddenly reminded of a small Baptist church in Alabama where—twenty-five years ago—I watched the black woman who was mother to me that summer "get happy with the Spirit," yelling, shrieking, and finally—restrained by the ushers—passing out on the floor. Now that the cousins have her firmly pinioned between them, Denise is free to flail wildly until she, too, seems to enter a trance and settles, with only a few spasmodic twitches, into a front row pew. That Denise—herself a severe and practicing alcoholic—is the one to wail the loudest is, I suppose, predictable. Bruce and she had earlier fought acrimoniously, but they had had no contact with each other for years.

The silence is once again broken by the processional, a loud, joyful song, accompanied, even, by a tambourine. It's been a long time since I've been to a funeral—never, I think, in a Roman Catholic church—so I initially find such a high spirited song at this time of mourning incongruous. Bruce did not have much: an abused childhood, twenty years of adulthood spent either drunk or in prison, and then eighteen months ago a diagnosis of AIDS. But this last year has had its share of joy, and he would have been the first to say so.

The certainty of premature death had given Bruce a reason to live fully the time he had remaining. He gave up his wine, although (I'd just found out) he had not given up his cocaine entirely. For the last year he has lived with us at Joseph's House. Claudia told me last week—after Bruce entered the hospital and drifted into coma, and I was trying to prepare Claudia and her sister Jeanne for Bruce's death—that she had never seen Bruce as happy as he had been during his time in Joseph's House. And my friendship with him has certainly been an unforgettable experience. The joyousness of the Catholic hymn quickly seems appropriate, and soon I join in the clapping. After all these years in the African American community, it finally seems natural to clap on the second and fourth beats of a measure.

Father Anderson moves easily into the comforting liturgy. A tall, ascetic-appearing white man in his fifties with long, bony fingers, he seems now, as always, a little nervous. Father Anderson had visited the shelter in which Bruce had lived for several months before coming to Joseph's House, and the two had become acquainted. Twice a year Father Anderson still says mass at the shelter for those who have "passed." He visits the living on a regular, weekly basis, more often when needed. Even his nervousness, the fact that one is never quite at ease in his presence, the fact that he never quite belongs to the people he has chosen as his own, signals something of his spirit and his compassion. I am not surprised Bruce chose him as pastor and teacher.

During the homily, I am grateful Father Anderson does not try to cast Bruce as a saint. We all know he drank and drugged the best years of his life away, that he abandoned his family, that he had killed a man, maybe two, that he could, at times, lash out viciously . . . even toward those he was close to. But Father Anderson reminds us of the value of all human life, reminds us of the many times Bruce did struggle to be good, reminds us of this last eighteen months of sobriety, his recent baptism, his desire to create something better.

Joseph's House is an eleven-bed home and community for homeless men with AIDS founded in 1990. A group of us formed a small non-profit organization and purchased a large, single-family dwelling in the Adams-Morgan neighborhood of Washington, D.C. Bruce was one of three men who lived with us during our first year while we awaited renovations that would make it possible for us to welcome our full complement of eleven men.

HIV infection among the homeless was already well established in 1990, but the first cases of full-blown AIDS were just showing up on the street and in my clinic, about a mile from Joseph's House. It was easy to predict that there would soon be many homeless men and women struggling with the weakness, intermittent illness, dementia, and hopelessness of this disease at the same time they had no place to call home, no place they could even retreat to on those days when they needed to rest or, perhaps, had an especially bad case of diarrhea. We wanted Joseph's House to be some small expression of hope.

Mostly, though, Marja and I and our children wanted to live in community with these men. We had worked with the poor long enough, lived long enough in their neighborhoods, tried long enough to establish relationships through our work—Marja as a teacher, I as a physician—but something always held me, at least, back. Always the distance between my life and theirs seemed unbridgeable. But although the intimate relationships I had desired never quite happened, my experiences had created within me the desire for a deeper life with people who had been excluded by the wider society. Would it be possible to become—in the usual sense of the word—"friends" or even "family"? In our eight years in Washington, the promise of community with the poor had not yet materialized. Perhaps Joseph's House would be an opportunity for a different kind of togetherness.

The first few weeks Bruce (nobody called him "Dennis," just "Bruce"), Ron, and Howard almost tiptoed around the house. They were not quite sure what the catch was. Was this simply another way station for them, another shelter—nicely appointed but still a shelter that would send them packing in a few weeks or a few months? It took some time for them to realize that Joseph's House was their home and that they could (and would, it turned out) stay with us until they died.

The three men were wildly different from one another. While on the streets, Howard had supported his drug addiction by burglarizing homes. He had been a "cat burglar," specializing in breaking into houses where the occupants were home and sleeping. But he had had a religious conversion. After he had been discovered to be HIV-positive and then hospitalized with brain damage, he was eventually discharged to Mother Teresa's Gift of Peace, a hospice for the destitute dying, some with AIDS, some with cancer, some with other terminal diseases. One day while reading a plaque listing all of the people who had died there, Howard suddenly saw his entire life differently. Realizing he had wasted his own life, he figured that whatever remaining life he had belonged to God. He began helping out, trying to be of service to the other residents. He discovered a unique gift in helping people move through their last hours: He would hold them, bathe them, clean them, feed them—whatever was needed. After some months, his health improved so much he no longer belonged in a hospice and was anxious to move with us into Joseph's House. But he continued to return two or three times a week to Gift of Peace to minister to the needs of homeless men who, like himself, were dying of AIDS.

Befitting his former profession, I suppose, Howard is a night owl. Most nights he stays up until six or seven in the morning, prowling the house. Sometimes when I cannot sleep, I come downstairs and find him at prayer in the living room. He says he spends about two hours before his homemade altar every night, a Baptist praying his rosary before the Holy Mother. During the other hours of the night, he finishes the dishes, cleans the kitchen, washes the floors, hooks someone's TV up to cable, and—during the summer—does the gardening and lawn work. But sometimes late at night he needs to talk about what it is like to work with people dying of the disease from which he himself will die, what it is like to change their bedpans and feed them, knowing that he might come to need the same help. And so we talk for an hour or so, a conversation that would never take place in an office or during a weekly counseling session.

Ron is the gregarious one in the house: pleasant and outgoing, always ready with a friendly word, always ready to stop and chat with whoever drops by. He has become very active in AA and NA, trying to lead others into recovery from drugs. He himself leads a twelve-step group for people with HIV infection, which met weekly for a while at the house. He has, even while sick with AIDS and living at Joseph's House, struggled with his addiction, several times relapsing back into using cocaine. It is from Ron that I have learned the awesome power of drug addiction and have been inspired by the courage of those who, while terminally ill with AIDS, nevertheless rise daily to fight the awful demon.

But there was always a special relationship between Bruce and me. He was a hardened street person, yet, at the very same time, there could be a little-boy innocence about him. He never knew his father, and his mother died when he was young. He moved in with his grandmother and was raised by two uncles who physically abused him. He was, he told me, beaten at least daily with a belt. Finally, at the age of seventeen, his uncle came at him one more time, and Bruce shot and killed him. From then on, he was in and out of reform schools and prisons, drinking as much as he could whenever he could. At one point during his years in prison he was put in solitary confinement ("the hole"), which he described to me.

"It's a cement room ten feet by ten feet. But it's only shoulder high, so you can't ever stand up straight. The only light is from the barred window at the door, so it's dark inside. There's no furniture, nothin'. They bring in a mattress at five in the evenin' and take it back out at five the next mornin'. They take all your clothes, so you're in there naked. In the corner is a hole in the cement which you're supposed to use as a toilet; they flush it every three days. There's one real meal every three days; the other times you just get a liquid stuff, sometimes enough, sometimes not, depending on their mood. Then every third day they take you out for a few minutes over to the doctor's who makes sure you're OK. Then they take you back. You've counted all the bricks by the end of the first day; there's not much else to do." Bruce once spent ninety days in a single stretch in the hole. "It's better than bein' on the bus," he said with resignation. "If they send you on the bus, you travel for months around the country from one federal prison to the other. The windows is all blacked out; it's dark and you can't see nothin'." The bus, apparently, takes prisoners from one prison to the other, but *is* the jail for some.

What amazes me is the lack of bitterness, the gentleness, and the humor with which he tells the story. Yet Bruce could be nasty to those he decided he did not like. Although he denied it when I asked him straight out, he certainly never liked Marja. Usually he would ignore her, pretending not to hear, not responding to her greeting, not answering her most innocuous questions. Those few times he would talk to her directly, he called her "Miss Marja," emphasizing, I suppose, his distance, his lack of intimacy, referring by implication to the centuries of black oppression.

Bruce knew Marja was thrifty, concerned not only with wastefulness but also with the ecological costs of expending nonrenewable resources. So when she was around, he seemed to take perverse pleasure in turning on the gas stove long before he was ready to put his bacon or his eggs on to fry. He was "just getting ready," he said. Marja would come into the kitchen, ask who left the gas on, and Bruce would continue as if he hadn't heard. He would open the refrigerator door, take out the bacon, eggs, vegetable oil, retrieve his spices from the cupboard, and beat his eggs; sometimes he would pour his juice or put his coffee on. Marja would ask, a little louder, "Who left the gas on?"

"I got ears," he would say stonily and turn coldly away. And then just as Marja was about to explode, he would turn the flame down and begin his bacon.

I once asked him directly what was wrong between him and Marja. Why did he not like her? He seemed honestly surprised. "Sure, I like her. She's an OK lady. I just talk trash a lot, Dr. David. There ain't nothin' between me and her. You got to understand, I just talk trash a lot." I could not bring myself to believe him, for I had watched him often enough with her, but was it possible that he was not really aware of his true feelings? I did not know.

But interrupting even his most abusive self, his deepest pain, was a smile, an innocence, a simplicity that attracted me. I once suggested a trip to visit Luray Caverns, and his face lit up with the delight of a child. When we went as a group to the circus, Bruce made a point of inviting a four-year-old boy whom he had known from his days on North Capitol Street. The boy was quiet, deferential, scared—quite clearly abused himself, which may have explained the depth of the relationship between him and Bruce. Bruce showed a boyish joyfulness in the simple things: an opportunity to help with shopping, a chance to go on a trip out of town, a word of approval. I will never forget his grin when he was happy. Even with his missing upper four front teeth, there was no mistaking the emotion!

In August of 1990, several months after he had come to Joseph's House, Bruce developed fever and shortness of breath. Because we had established connections with the AIDS clinic at Georgetown University Hospital, Bruce was admitted without delay to the doctors who knew him and his medical condition. He became gravely ill with *Pneumocystis Carinii* pneumonia, a potentially fatal complication of AIDS. But Bruce had the best medical care and by the fourth day was improving. A week later he was discharged. We brought him home with us and watched him carefully.

Within twenty-four hours, however, Bruce had gone back to bed, lying alone in his room, weak, confused, and listless. He did not want help, he said, but I knew that something was very wrong. We took him back to the emergency room where the examining doctor believed the problem to be dehydration and sent Bruce back home. But it was obvious to us who knew him so well that something more significant than dehydration was going on.

The next morning we took him a second time to the emergency room, and this time he was admitted. Addison's Disease, an unusual hormonal deficiency sometimes associated with AIDS, had developed and seriously threatened his life. The problem was diagnosed, Bruce was treated appropriately, and within a few days he was back home with us. But what would have happened if he had originally been discharged to a shelter rather than Joseph's House? His sleepiness and listlessness would almost certainly been interpreted as intoxication. He would most likely have died then and there.

I felt grateful for Joseph's House.

AIDS can cause a kind of senility, "AIDS dementia," which manifests itself as a difficulty remembering, a lessening of judgment, an inability to think clearly. Bruce certainly suffered from this complication. Because of his years of alcohol abuse, it was difficult to know what was AIDS dementia, what was brain damage from the alcohol, and what was just Bruce's contrariness. But as the year progressed, he deteriorated. Around Christmastime, Bruce had to be hospitalized once again for an infection. As he was recuperating, he became upset with the confinement and—with his lightning quick temper—became verbally abusive with the nurses who were caring for him. The resident doctor called me at Joseph's House. Because of his behavior Bruce was being discharged from the hospital and would not be welcome back at the AIDS clinic or in the hospital.

Bruce recovered from the infection, but his expulsion from the clinic seemed to me a potential disaster. After what I'd seen in my ten years of practicing in the community, I did not want to trust him to the public clinics. I knew how important it was for him to see doctors who knew him, to have the continuity of care anyone deserves.

"I know I shouldn't a-done it, Dr. David. It wasn't her fault, the nurse. I get to talkin' trash and they don't know I don't mean nothin' by it. But she kept comin' in when I was asleep and puttin' that needle in my arm or takin' my blood pressure without even askin'. You got to wake a man up an' tell him what you're doin'."

I had watched medical personnel try to do their jobs on sleeping patients, and I presumed the nurse was only doing her best. But she apparently did not realize that one does not approach homeless men while they are asleep to do *anything* to them: too much happens to sleeping men on the street, and they have been conditioned. We had learned at home to tap Bruce on the feet and wait until he was fully awake before doing anything.

Bruce was divided. On the one hand, he knew that he had overreacted to whatever had been inconsiderate in the nurse's response to his needs; on the other hand, he was not really capable of talking about it without getting angry all over again. As we talked with him, we realized that Bruce had never really learned to apologize. So we coached him, working with him on just what to say, helping him make an appointment with the nurse, accompanying him as he went over to apologize.

He came home with that wide, toothless yet paradoxically boyish grin. "I did it!" he whooped. "I told her I didn't mean nothin' by it, and she said it was OK."

The nurse talked with the doctor, and by Christmas Bruce was reinstated at the clinic.

I found myself learning continuously from Bruce, learning to value the life I'd been given, learning to value the little things that made each day worthwhile. In the world's terms, Bruce had little. He had accomplished little, had few relationships, had little to look forward to. He had few of those internal reserves that most of us create out of those experiences of being loved and cared for, so there was little with which to deal with the coming adversity. In spite of it, however, Bruce made a decision for life, decided to live as fully as he could with the time he had left.

He and I talked from time to time of his impending death. He did not want anyone to pull the plug, no matter what the prognosis, he said; he wanted all possible medical treatment. Since virtually every other man in Joseph's House has since requested that hopeless treatment not be continued, I now believe that Bruce's decision was motivated at least in part by his inability to trust that anyone else would really make decisions in his best interest. But his decision also indicated how much he cared for his life, as limited as it was.

Bruce's terminal illness went quickly. Except for an intermittent fever persistent over months (for which neither I nor the specialists had been able to find the cause), I had no hint of his terminal condition until his roommate Ron found him one late-May morning, incoherent and incontinent in bed. He had soiled his clothes, the sheets, and himself with diarrhea. I was grateful for Howard's abilities learned at Gift of Peace. While I ran to the drugstore for an adult-sized diaper, Howard cleaned Bruce off and began cleaning up the worst of the mess in the room.

When I returned, Howard helped me dress Bruce, and together we jack-knifed him into the car.

Just before we drove off, Howard handed me a small pipe, used for smoking cocaine, that he had found while removing the dirty linen for washing. Driving Bruce to the hospital and waiting with him as he sank deeper into coma, I had a chance to reflect on the meaning of the pipe.

In retrospect, we had been incredibly naive. Both Lois, the nurse who lived with us, and I had had significant experience working with inner-city people with severe addictions. We were aware of how manipulative and secretive people with addictions could be; nevertheless, we thought that living with a person on a day-to-day basis we would be able to tell before he had relapsed very far back into his addiction. Six months before, we had found a similar cocaine pipe in the pocket of an overcoat that Bruce had recently acquired at a nearby clothes closet for the homeless. We allowed Bruce and Ron to convince us that the pipe must have been in the pocket before Bruce acquired it. It wasn't much of an excuse, but I guess we just did not want to see what was right before our noses. This new concrete evidence helped me to understand that we had been willing to ignore a number of behavioral changes over the spring months. Bruce, and probably Ron, had been using for months. Only much later could we pin Ron down and deal with the problem.

Bruce had told me that he wanted his family notified if "things look bad," and now they did. I called his sister Claudia. Bruce had not had much to do with his family during most of adulthood, but in the last year he had made contact with Claudia and begun to talk also with Jeanne. I tried to set up a time to meet with the two sisters together, but each kept asking me to be the one to talk to the other and find a common time. It soon became apparent that neither sister was, for whatever reason, talking to the other.

I pushed ahead anyway, and one Monday evening both sisters came over to Joseph's House. I explained the situation, making reference to his AIDS. Jeanne was shocked since Bruce had never told her of his diagnosis. We talked of his year in Joseph's House, and both sisters reaffirmed its importance to Bruce. We talked about the likelihood of his death, and there were tears. By the end of the evening, the sisters—who hadn't talked with one another in over a year—were holding each other and crying. In his death, at least, Bruce was bringing his family together.

Once in the hospital, Bruce roused temporarily, and—although they still had no idea what had caused his collapse—the doctors were even thinking of sending him back home. But, as quickly as the last time, he slipped into coma and—despite all his doctors could do—died of what turned out on autopsy to be an abdominal infection.

In the last days of his life at the hospital, Bruce's doctors told us that he stood no chance of survival. But, since Bruce had been unwilling to give any-one power of medical attorney, "treatment" continued while the hospital did tests to determine whether he was "brain dead," which would give them the legal authority to turn off the machines without permission. We were told that the final determination would be made at 5:00 P.M. on a Wednesday, so all of us from his "family" at Joseph's House packed into cars and drove to the hospital to be present. There were, perhaps, ten of us circled around Bruce's bed, waiting, wanting both to be there and far away. But the attending physi-cian never showed, the "pulling of the plug" was postponed, and Bruce's body gave out of its own within twenty-four hours.

After the homily, Father Anderson invites us all to share our remembrances of Bruce's life. Taking our cue from the priest, none of us seems to need to make Bruce into a saint, either, yet each of us has seen something of God in Bruce. Despite his abuse towards her, Marja remembers his boyish smile and the joy he took in taking his little friend to the circus. Sr. Lenora—the nurse from the shelter who had been so close to him, visiting almost every day, shepherding him through the classes for baptismal candidates—remembers his desire for baptism and his discipline in coming to the weekly classes.

One of the older men sitting outside the pillar stands unsteadily and be-gins a meandering monologue. He is obviously drunk, but he, too, wants to pay his respects to Bruce. He knows also, he says, how important this past year at Joseph's House was to Bruce. "He liked that place up there. He still came down to sit with us, but he wasn't drinkin'. He just come down and sit with us, and I'd go get him a soda, and he'd drink his soda while the rest of us were drinkin'." He stands unsteadily. I cannot understand most of his slurred speech, but he continues speaking for some minutes, trying to articulate the value of his relationship with his dead friend, reemphasizing almost with awe that Bruce did not drink when he came down to North Capitol.

I look around the sanctuary at this unusual expression of community. It is,

I realize suddenly, what I have come to the inner city for, what I have been looking for these many years. In front of me is his family, finally gathered together in his death. The formerly estranged sisters, Claudia and Jeanne, are weeping in each other's arms. To one side are his friends from the shelter, friends who have also at one time lived on the street. Over there are those middle-class people from my faith community who, like myself, have been in one way or another friend to Bruce. And we are all listening with some patience to the rambling eulogy for a street person by an intoxicated street person. In the entire scheme of things, nothing terribly important happened at Joseph's House this past year. The awful oppression under which the poor suffer has scarcely been alleviated by our work. The political conditions that formed the backdrop of Bruce's unhappy life are unchanged by the experience of the past year. And yet Bruce has brought us together—rich and poor, black and white, powerful and powerless—in order to remember him. He has created of us—if only for a moment—a form of community. It is the desire for this community that has brought me to the inner city.

Have a Beautiful Day Hot Air Balloons

L. J. Schneiderman

Old Uncle Sam—I can still hear my father's ironic mockery every time I say his name—Uncle Sam likes when I set him where he can watch the hot air balloons. A company called "Have a Beautiful Day Hot Air Balloons" launches tourists and conventioneers from the beach. As the balloons catch the evening breeze and rise over the park, you can hear the roar of the torch and see the faces of the people in the bannered gondolas.

"Have a Beautiful Day," the baskets cheerfully command.

Mr. Do, from the nursing home, and I sit on a bench alongside the wheelchair. The kids in the park, mostly Vietnamese like Mr. Do, will wave to the people overhead, and if they wave back, the kids shriek and laugh and fall all over each other.

The ocean is a dull pewter, as though the low sunlight has skimmed off its sheen, the balloons radiant in the last broadside. Some Sundays as many as a dozen or so, striped and spiral-colored, fill the sky. We follow them as they float over the rumbling interstate freeway and broad lagoon of clay tile roofs toward the mountains, gradually shrinking into drops of wine that slide down into the burgundy haze.

"You think he's comfortable?" I always ask.

"Oh, yes," Mr. Do always answers.

Somehow he manages to get my uncle into a grey suit and polished loafers, a handkerchief fluffed in his breast pocket. Under his baseball cap a twist of mouth, a smile actually.

"Happy? Really happy?"

"Oh, yes. Very happy."

I watch as Mr. Do pulls out Uncle Sam's handkerchief and wipes his face. Like a bird brushing about a piece of garden statuary.

I remember I am—what?—four, perhaps five years old, looking up at this strange man swabbing his bald head, embracing a brown paper bag. Jacket and pants droop in mismatched patterns of grey. Even that child could recognize they come from different suits. The man gives his mouth a strange twist of a smile. "Not something you expect to find on your doorstep, am I?"

"This is your Uncle Sam," my father says, without looking at either of us.

That night at dinner he asks me, "So what do you want to be when you grow up, young man?" digging the words out of his throat the way my father does. It's not the slurring effortless speech I hear from everyone else—like warm sand running through your fingers—and I realize for the first time that my father too comes from another place.

"A doctor," I say.

The man looks at my father. "You see. It runs in the family."

My father's gruff answer surprises me. "So what does that make me—the family idiot?"

Later I hear them downstairs. "Everyone has troubles," my father rages. Look what happened to *him*—he had to drop his used car business and scramble to find work at Convair. Otherwise it was the army! Even though he had a kid! Just when business was picking up! Whole trainloads of families arriving every day to be near their men in uniform. Willing to pay *anything*. And now the damn blackout in case of Japanese bombers. What did H. V. Kaltenborn call them? Yellow Peril! *Orientals!* Not even human.

I creep to the window, terrified that I might see oriental submarines rising from the moon-glittering water; then creep back to my bed and, while they continue quarreling, lie there in the dark listening to the radio, hearing my father's taunts through the music.

"So, what did you expect from your little brother, Uncle Sam? What do you expect from the family idiot?"

"He doesn't even go to Hebrew school."

"Here nobody speaks Hebrew!"

"When he grows up, what will he be?"

"Smarter than you, Uncle Sam. Bet on it!"

Until he could pass an exam and practice medicine again, Uncle Sam went to work selling cars, filling in during my father's shift at Convair. I remember seeing him there—bobbing around the lot behind the darting strides of my father, trying to pick up sales techniques, such as letting a customer take a car home for a few days before paying for it. ("Watch the eyes. Some people you do them a favor, they're hooked.")

A disaster.

"The Ford coupe with leatherette covers, Uncle Sam! The Plymouth with only three thou on it. Where'd they go?"

"People cheat. What can I do?"

"The eyes," I said, "watch their *eyes*."

But Uncle Sam found no answers in the eyes.

Night after night contempt and exasperation boil up in my father's voice, usually ending with his providing a longer list—brothers and sisters, aunts, uncles, cousins, all of them professors, doctors, bigshots as fancy and distinguished as Uncle Sam pretended to be—all named with a vengeance. Why didn't he go to *them* for help?

Gently, always gently, Uncle Sam reminds him they are all gone.

"So? So? You should have left when the family idiot did!" And a door would slam.

And I would hear Uncle Sam acknowledge in the silence that yes, his little brother had outsmarted them all.

The night before Uncle Sam moves out, the mild-mannered man finally lets his temper fly. I hold my breath at what I hear. *Shit for brains!* Did he think he hadn't *tried* to get out? Their old father stubborn . . . mother hopeless . . . the children. . . . *He at least remembered his responsibilities!* They got as far as Paris, where the police—the *police,* no less!—grabbed their papers and ordered them into a huge stadium that was used for bicycle races. Separated into long lines, and made to stand for hours. Thousands of people. Just before she was taken away, Moira, his daughter, begs him, "Why must I do this? Haven't I been a good girl?"

I don't remember the answer Uncle Sam gave to his daughter. I was busy picturing the scene—shaping it from the lights cast on the ceiling by my radio. A huge stadium just for bicycle races!

My father had started taking me to high school football games. People shouting, waving flags, singing, while bands played and cheerleaders jumped and did cartwheels and pyramids, my father never failing to point out to me his advertisement in the program they gave out. It had a picture of a soldier and sailor carrying American flags.

By the time I returned to Uncle Sam's story, he was packed in a truck with other men. The truck broke down and the men had to march to a train. Along the way people jeering. My father protests. He doesn't want to hear these things! "You will hear these things!" Uncle Sam shouts. He pauses for breath. "We get to a station. A huge crowd now." Each sentence is like a massive door Uncle Sam has to push open. "We're standing around. Waiting. And all of a sudden. I take one little step. To the side. Like this. That's all, just like this"—his voice made an odd squeak—"and I start jeering, too. And that's how I got left behind. I became one of them. One of those people."

Even from my bed I could tell what his face looked like, his strange twist of a smile.

"You'll see. Now you'll be rich," was all my father said. "Here all the doctors are rich."

And that was the last I saw of Uncle Sam until the synagogue from L.A.

called me. Their computer system had sounded the alert. He was delinquent on his pledge. I was listed on his file card. Did I know anything about it? A doctor, too. Usually they're so reliable.

Mr. Do gets up and adjusts Uncle Sam's baseball cap, which keeps sliding to the side. He leans over to hoist him up in the wheelchair. The two men embrace, look briefly at each other—a smile—then Mr. Do sits back down. We continue to gaze at the balloons and the blue-shadowed waves of mountains beyond them.

I realize I am touched by the way Mr. Do hugged my uncle. "You miss your home?" I ask. It is the first time I venture a personal question.

Mr. Do shrugs.

The lightness of the gesture takes me by surprise, offends me. Is that it? The Vietnam War—a *shrug!*

And my response surprises me, too. It is almost a lunge, a physical bursting out of long-buried resentment. Has he already forgotten, I hear myself scolding him. The victims. Not only his Vietnamese people and our American soldiers, the dead and maimed. Others he probably did not even know about. Those of us who fought against the war back home. Crippled by rashly made choices. Prison. Canada. All of us stuck in a charred bitterness that cannot be scoured. So much hate in this country now, unforgotten, unforgiven, and I hear myself go on at length about how I had marched and demonstrated, how I had screwed up my chance of tenure and broke with my woman, and yes, spent a night in jail.

Mr. Do does not seem exactly swept away by my lament. And in fact I am annoyed at myself for being so provoked by his shrug. His smile remains blandly unmoved, a geisha smile, hands folded in his lap.

"So," I ask, impatiently, but determined to be tolerant, "what did you do in Vietnam?" He had been the enemy after all, the side I had been demonstrating against. I try to engage his eyes.

"Doctor."

"Doctor. No kidding?" I am surprised, actually. And I let my voice rise to signify that I'm impressed. "No kidding." I nod in the direction of Uncle Sam. "So was he, you know?"

Mr. Do nods. He knows.

"You knew that?"

"Oh, yes."

"How about you?" I ask. "You hoping to practice again someday?"

"Oh, yes," Mr. Do nods.

"You'll have to take some kind of test."

"Yes. Take test."

Though he can barely speak English he makes it seem so easy. Yet I think what magic these little people possess, the tricks they can do. Everywhere you look you find them, their children, barely settled in and already winning spelling bees and scholarships, flooding libraries and laboratories, making Phi Beta Kappa and Westinghouse Honor Roll.

"That's what he had to do," I say. "Take some kind of test."

Mr. Do smiles blandly, nods.

I describe how while waiting to take the test for a medical license, Old Uncle Sam also had to do other work to support himself. He tried selling cars. I laugh at the memory. Then I become embarrassed by the sound of my voice, the echo of my father's contempt for the lofty doctor's humiliation.

Is Mr. Do offended? His eyes are resting peacefully on the balloons, which are miles away now, no more than festive ornaments hanging in the sky.

"How did you manage to get out?"

Silence.

Then I heard the word.

"Boat."

He accompanied it with the briefest twist of a smile.

So, he was one of the famous boat people. Not so long ago—when was it?—they too had their fifteen minutes, their headlines and feature stories, their television specials. Overloaded hulks. Thai pirates. Rapings, lootings, murder. I look at him closely. Could this delicate creature have endured anything as terrible as that?

"What was it like?" I said, meaning, of course, what was it really like.

Mr. Do smiled. "Boat sank."

"How then . . . ?"

He shrugged. "Lucky." Again that smile.

"It helps to be lucky, doesn't it?"

He nodded.

"Some people weren't so lucky, I suppose."

He nodded.

"Who? People you knew?"

Again a silence. Then the words.

"Wife. Children."

It was my turn to be silent. I couldn't speak. As though my mouth were filled with shattered glass.

Meanwhile, around me, the world carried on as usual. The balloons now dotted the sky in colorful musical notation, like a jaunty Sousa march. Uncle Sam was smiling at the children cheerfully and indignantly squirting water at each other from the fountain.

"He lost his family too," I said finally, trying to make up for my clumsiness.

"I know."

"What? What do you know," I demanded.

The answer scratched against my face. And for a man who must never in his life have heard a remotely similar concatenation of sounds, he pronounced it perfectly.

"Auschwitz."

And just then I heard the spurting noise, turbulent and urgent. Right over our heads. Another balloon. Massively alone and seemingly crippled. Apparently it had gotten off late and was in trouble, its torch sputtering on and off.

When the children on the ground caught sight of the struggling beast they went wild with laughter. They had never seen anything so hilarious. In the gondola were four or five children, waving uncertainly. You could tell by the way they clung to the wicker sides that they were waving to cover their fear.

"Have a Beautiful Day," said the flapping red, white, and blue banner.

Again and again the torch snorted and the huge shape undulated protestingly, like some thick liquid trying to dissolve.

Uncle Sam's wheelchair creaked, and I became aware that he was grunting and twisting. He seemed to be in pain.

"Mr. Do," I said.

The dainty geisha man leaned over, listened, then smiled and nodded and gave him a gentle pat.

"What? What's he saying?"

Still smiling Mr. Do looked up, shrugged.

"He say, 'Get out.'"

Now the children were cheering. The balloon was struggling to make its way to the Kmart parking lot just across the freeway. With each desperate gasp it sank lower and lower over the speeding cars, its torch snorting convulsively. It managed to stay aloft just long enough to reach the edge of the tarmac where it squatted with doddering relief. The neon bright fabric collapsed, enveloping the basket in one last display, like a peacock spreading its tail.

After a few moments we could see the children beating their way out from under it, flinging their arms and stomping triumphantly. They ran this way and that. I almost imagined I could hear their high-pitched voices, although at that distance and with so many other sounds—the cars, the ocean, the cheers of the children around me—I doubt it. And I caught something else, although I couldn't be sure of that either, again that smile—it passed between the two men.

"What?" I said to Mr. Do. But he didn't answer. Instead he was staring, both of them were staring, smiling, not at the balloon in the parking lot, but off into the distance at the other balloons, now small and insubstantial as bubbles, descending and one by one disappearing into the wine-dark haze.

Max and the Golden Mean

JACK COULEHAN

THE BEST WAY to understand how I felt about Max and her lung transplant is to tell you about the Golden Mean.

I'm a fanatic for balance. Harmony, balance, consensus, moderation. Not getting all riled up about taxes or politics. Homeostasis. Step by step. Self-correcting feedback. Taking the middle course. Being able to see the point in different points of view. You get the idea. When I was a kid, I never thought this attitude was surprising—it was me, after all—nor did I attribute it to star signs or horoscopes, items that didn't exist at all in my family, not even for fun. It must have been during high school that I learned I was a Libra, balance personified, and this was a burden. It was, after all, the Age of Aquarius, and I wanted desperately to be outrageous.

At the liberal arts college I attended, to graduate you had to take two courses in philosophy. One was Intro, which in my year was taught by Mr. Ryer because the priest who used to teach it had left the order. Mr. Ryer used to be a cab driver in New York and since then had been writing his book on Being. He would bring a stone into class and stand there with the stone in the palm of his hand and stare at it. He told us to stare at it, too. To try to get inside the stone, to experience "stone-ing," a process that involved screwing up our foreheads and glancing back and forth at the stapled mimeographed pages of chapter 3. Chapter 3 was the only part of the book on Being Mr. Ryer ever managed to complete, and it was utterly incomprehensible, not because the concepts were complicated but because they didn't make sense.

The second philosophy course was ethics, which was a heady mixture of Aristotle and St. Thomas Aquinas. The main thing that impressed me about Aristotle was the Golden Mean, the idea that virtue lies in the middle ground between two extremes. Take courage, for example. You have this continuum and at one end is spinelessness; at the other end is recklessness. Somewhere in between, at just the right place, where God or Aristotle had put it, lies courage the way it should be, steadfast without being rash or overbearing. Well, you get the idea. You can do this Golden Mean thing with other virtues, too, like prudence or magnanimity. I loved it.

My roommate, who was Italian and the funniest person I've ever known, absolutely refused to believe in the Golden Mean. Moderation, he said, is not a Mediterranean trait. He couldn't believe that the greatest of all Greek thinkers, a guy who worked obsessively, putting in maybe eighty hours a week inventing biology and categorizing the universe, could be dead wrong about moderation. Fred thought that Aristotle must have written a book about passion that was later suppressed by the Church. You've got Aristotle's *Ethics,* he said. And you've got *Poetics.* And *Politics.* And, for God's sake, *Metaphysics.* But somewhere there has to be a lost book, a lost key to wisdom. Imagine what we've been missing all these years. Could it be Aristotle's *Erotics?* Or the *Nicomachean Obsessives?* The way Fred went on riffs about Aristotle, you'd never believe that the Golden Mean wound up having such a lasting effect in his life. In fact, he became an endocrinologist and devoted his career to balancing hormones in Houston.

With me it was about the same, practicing general medicine. Getting up in the morning and balancing one thing or another—time, energy, interest, drugs, money, and hope. You name it. Not too much, not too little. It wore me down being moderate. But then Maxine O'Reilly came along.

One morning as I walked into her hospital room, Max thrust a page of the *Post Gazette* into my hands, and pulled off her Venti mask. "Whsssh . . ." said the oxygen.

"Take a look."

"Toss aside all thoughts of failure. Make a fresh start. Don't let others lead you astray."

"That's it," she said. "I'm Taurus the Bull. That's my horoscope."

Her small body was smudged with sweat and fever, but those eyes . . . Wow! And on a Monday morning, too. That's the first time she asked me about getting a lung transplant. I have to tell you it wasn't pleasant. In fact, I felt a kind of repulsion, as if Max and I were magnets approaching each other's positive pole. Yes, I wanted Max to live. I was invested in it. So much so that I imagined each setback reversible and her future a tolerable compromise with severely damaged lungs. But transplant? That seemed so drastic, so immoderate.

"What do you think, doc? Let's whip out the old and put in the new."

Some months earlier, Max had strode into my office unannounced while I was dictating the previous patient's note.

"Hi, doc. Are you ready for me? I'm Max."

She was a small woman, not yet forty, whose sharp tongue and angular features took her straight to the point. Her problem was a condition called bronchiectasis, which had gradually destroyed her lungs through repeated infection. "I just can't clear the goop, that's the long and short of it," she explained.

At that first visit she looked like a champ, but within a month she was down for the count. High fever, shaking cough, breathlessness. Full cups of brown sputum. Years of chronic infection had left her small bronchioles largely destroyed and their defenses nonexistent. However, after a few days in the hospital, as the intravenous antibiotics and steroids took hold, Max's condition improved. In a week or so, her nervous blue hands were back to folding origami. Max was a compulsive folder. Swans. Frogs. Deer. A hippopotamus.

"The hippo's for you," she told me. "Now, please, I've got to get out of this hospital before I go crazy."

Max's renaissance didn't last long. As soon as we stopped the antibiotics and tapered her steroid dosage, the fever and breathlessness returned. The small, charged body shrank to a core of night sweats, air hunger, rapid heartbeat, and hands grasping my wrist. But Max's eyes were defiant.

On antibiotics again, she softened and told me about growing up in McKees Rocks, where her violent, alcoholic father hustled votes for the Democratic machine, after he lost his job at the mill. He was a big, red-faced man whose motto was "Don't tread on me," though he must have known enough to realize the bosses walked all over him and there was nothing he could do about it. After he died, Max's mother made do by cleaning other people's houses. She and the girls. There were four girls, Max the oldest. Max's break came when the nuns got her a scholarship to a Catholic women's college far enough away that she couldn't go home on weekends.

Before I knew her, Max worked as a counselor at an alcohol rehabilitation program. A recovering alcoholic, she was proud of her nine years without a drink. One day at a time. Alcohol had almost killed her. Once, in a drunken stupor on the sidewalk in front of her apartment house, she had been forced to roll against the concrete steps and pull herself up by the iron filigree of the banister. The next day she began to pull herself together. She joined Alcoholics Anonymous and somewhere along the line met Sam. Sam was the blind African American man who sat for hours each day beside Max's hospital bed, working furiously on his Braille laptop computer. He was a criminology professor at one of our local universities. He studied recidivism in prisoners. Whenever we had an opportunity to talk, I kept going back to recidivism. Why can't we rehabilitate the prisoner? What's the problem with criminal justice? Doesn't anything help? Sam told me it was complicated. When things were going poorly for Max, I learned to expect Sam's melodious bass voice in the background, "It's rough today, real rough, but we'll lick this yet."

Max and Sam: tough knocks.

A few days before Christmas, after several such cycles of renaissance and relapse, Maxine popped her magnetic question.

My first response was, "She's desperate. Someone has been filling her full of false hopes. I don't want to deal with this. Not today."

But why not? Let's take a look at the facts. Max was definitely going downhill, although the source of her problem was somewhat mysterious. It's not like she suffered from cystic fibrosis, a disease you can pinpoint right down to the enzyme. So what started the bronchiectasis ball rolling? None of the specialists could say. We searched the textbooks. Could it be something called impaired cilia syndrome? And why was it progressing despite the efforts of all the king's horses and all the king's men? In the absence of an enzyme or mechanism to blame, I created scenarios in which Max in a mysterious way finally avoided the precipice. Maybe the antibiotics would tip the balance. Maybe her immune system would marshal its forces and save the day. Lung transplantation, on the other hand, was far from imaginary. It was radical and risky. It represented a whole new world that I found alarming because Max would have to abandon the natural uncertainty of her future for the medicalized uncertainty of surgery, tissue rejection, and immune suppression. Transplantation had to be a false hope, I told myself. Yet, since every one of Max's options was fraught with uncertainty, why was I so reluctant?

Yet here was Max, my Max. I had grown to fancy myself as playing a role in her story. Sometimes my role was that of a wise magician, sometimes a friendly mechanic, and sometimes a deadpanning vaudevillian straight man. Now she wanted to bring in a new actor, a deus ex machina. How ungrateful, I thought. How immoderate! Poor Max, she doesn't understand that the god of the machine is likely to be a defective god.

"Well, we'll see," I told her. "It's something to consider."

A few days later, when a fellow from the transplant team took a look at Max, he went away shaking his head. Her outlook seemed very grim. To become a transplant candidate, she would have to overcome a number of hurdles, each of which was formidable. Her steroid dose was far too high and would need to be successfully tapered. She needed too much oxygen; somehow oxygen transport would have to improve. Likewise, the team couldn't begin to get serious unless Max's infection cleared. I tried my best to reassure her, while cautioning against false hope.

"After all," I said, "it's not like you need surgery any time soon. There's lots of room to maneuver, you know, we just have to find the right mixture . . ."

Her fingers were rapidly folding a swan. They stopped. She looked up. "A tough row to hoe," Max said. "Let's go for it. Let's do it."

We switched her to an aerosolized antibiotic that had recently been used with good results in cystic fibrosis patients, and then tapered her prednisone while adding a slew of aerosols and nebulizers.

I don't know how much to attribute to hope and how much to the new regimen, but Max blossomed. She went home from the hospital and stayed there. Thereafter, every few weeks she appeared in my office with a knapsack of oxygen, followed by Sam with his left hand on her shoulder and the computer in his briefcase. "Down to twenty milligrams," she would crow about the prednisone. And, after I congratulated her on the (relatively) clear chest, "How do you like those marbles?"

I still couldn't bring myself to be enthusiastic about the quest. After all, Max was unexpectedly improving on medical therapy. So, said the voice of moderation, maybe she won't need a new set of lungs. The Golden Mean would dictate that we harmonize, finesse, and stay put. I visualized the weeks of intense suffering she would be subjected to—the probing, the pain, the tubes, the outlandish infections. The surgeons and intensivists would turn Max into a challenge, a problem, a pincushion, an objet d'art. And what if she did survive? How likely was it that she would be able to lead a fuller, more active life than she did at present? In my story, Max was a chronically ill patient who ought to compress her life into the Fates' compartment. In her story, she was the queen of the swans.

In the midst of applying for Social Security on the basis of "total and permanent disability," Max told me about her goal of going back to work after the operation. "You don't have to walk too much as a counselor," she assured me. "And I can always sit down." Her image of the future had her re-employment scheduled shortly after a celebratory trip to Maui.

You might be surprised from what I've told you that during these months Max was often frightened. She'd get spells when anxiety tightened its hands on her throat and set off spasms of labored breathing. Sam had trouble distinguishing these panic attacks from the breathlessness of new infection. So did I. He'd call me, sometimes late at night, and we'd agonize together over whether to send her to the emergency room, or try a relaxation tape that might allow her to sleep.

As far as I can tell, Max believed in horoscopes only when they worked to her advantage or when she could kid me about being a Libra. It's obvious, she announced, that thoughtfulness and balance are excellent traits in a doctor. But they do tend to make a man less interesting. "That's okay," she told me. "I can stand the boredom." Max also liked the way I usually saw her on time (unlike many of her doctors), but she hoped that moderation didn't interfere with my sense of humor. To be helpful, Max would clip my horoscope for the day to share during her office visits.

Someone wants to put the blame on you. Protect your interests. Let it be known that you will fight if the cause is right. ["Watch your ass," she told me.]

Lie low, play a waiting game. Legal ramifications have yet to be understood. ["I'm on your side. Let me take the witness stand."]

New faces and new vistas are around the next corner. Follow your instincts. Others accuse you of being opportunistic. ["What's your secret, doc?"]

By September Maxine had graduated to become a full-fledged lung transplant candidate. Shortly thereafter, I moved to another city, but asked Max and Sam to keep me up to date about how things were going. The first I heard from them, two or three months later, was a delighted phone call from Disney World.

"This isn't Maui," Max said, "and I don't have the new lungs, but here I am." My patient and her blind consort had achieved one of their goals, a vacation in Fantasyland. It must have been quite a production. I could imagine the oxygen apparatus, the nebulizers, the special accommodations. How did the two of them get around? Stop it, I told myself. The Magic Kingdom is magic. At least they'll have the trip to remember.

That's the thing—I could appreciate Max's passion when it came to thumbing her nose at the world, as long as it didn't involve my view of the world.

A winter passed. Then spring. One night in June the telephone awakened me. It was Sam. They had found a pair of lungs for Maxine, the lungs of a thirteen-year-old girl killed that day in an automobile accident. Max was in surgery that very minute. They wanted me to know. I muttered a few words of support, but later in my dream saw Max disappear into what looked like a Tunnel of Love, but within the tunnel were mechanical arms that began to grab her from all sides and, bit by bit, to tear her apart. This is the beginning of the end, I thought, and made a mental note to call her in a few days. But the mental note got lost. It was a busy week. The following week was busier yet. Mostly, I avoided calling because I didn't want to have to listen to Sam's sad voice describing in his meticulous way what Max was going through. A few weeks later, I did send a get-well note with a pop-out koala bear. That way, I reasoned, Max and Sam will know that I'm thinking of them.

In another week or so, my phone rang. "I'm calling about a breath of fresh air," a voice said. "Got your note, but I've been busy."

It was Max. Her familiar wheeze was gone, as was the "whsssh" of oxygen behind each sentence. She had returned home from the hospital the week earlier, feeling strong and unscathed after a merely "normal" complement of setbacks, including a "teeny" bout of cytomegalovirus pneumonia.

"I went to Sam's office for a couple of hours today, just to help out," she reported. "Filed a few papers. Didn't get winded, though. But, doc, here's what I wanted to tell you. Remember the first time you told me that I ought to consider a lung transplant? Well, I was scared to death. When you said the word 'transplant', I thought it was all over for me. So did Sam. I didn't know what to do. I didn't know how I could make it. But you kept us going, doc. You stuck with us. So I just wanted to say thanks for all your help."

Thanks for my help? I took a deep breath and said, "Max . . ."

The next morning I checked my horoscope in *Newsday*. "Let go of preconceived notions," it said. "Emphasize independence, originality. Make a fresh start in a new direction." I don't want to make too much of this, but the more you think about it, the more you realize that the Golden Mean has limits. Take compassion, for example, or joy or gratitude. Or better yet, take love. Where do you draw the line when it comes to love? Is love best when it's a balanced and comfortable kind of love? When it fits in and doesn't make waves? That's a good question. And I'm sure Max has a good answer.

Tara Sunshine

Fitzhugh Mullan

TARA SUNSHINE WAS her name. Tara Sunshine Smith. Dr. Milton liked her immediately. For a five-year-old she was very self-possessed. "My name is Tara Sunshine," she told him in the examination room. "This is my mother. Her name is Bright Sunshine. I was born Tara Sunshine, but her name used to be Nancy. She changed it before I was born."

"I see," said Dr. Milton. The girl was dressed in a faded, long dress that showed no signs of a recent washing. She wore sandals without socks, although the month was November. A small peace sign pendant hung from a lanyard around her neck. Her most striking feature was a head of lush blond hair that she wore in pigtails clipped at the ends with unmatched barrettes. "Mommy brought me because my ear hurts. It really hurts a lot," Tara went on.

"Doctor, we don't usually use doctors," Bright Sunshine explained, "but Tara's ear has been hurting for a week. Even though Seneca didn't want us to come, I thought we'd better."

"Who's Seneca?" Dr. Milton inquired.

"Seneca. Seneca Smith. My husband, her dad. You see we're independent people, and we don't really believe in Western medicine. You know what I mean?"

Dr. Milton knew what she meant. He worked at the People's Doctor, the only clinic in the Santa Fe area that treated all comers—the permanently poor, the temporarily poor, migrants, transients, legals, and illegals. Most of Dr. Milton's patients were the working poor, largely Hispanic people whose ancestors had lived in northern New Mexico since well before it belonged to the United States. Santa Fe was also a magnet for the counterculture—travelers from the East and West, flower people, herbalists, collectivists, dope heads, and nonconformists of every creed. Variable as their philosophies were, most of these people had in common an absence of health insurance and a lack of money. Many frequented the People's Doctor and Dr. Milton.

"I'm not sure what we want to do about it," said Bright Sunshine. "But I'd like you to take a look and tell me what you think is wrong." She was a tall woman with an angular face, a similarly dirty floor-length, patchwork dress, complicated hoop earrings, and multiple bracelets on both wrists. She smelled of damp wood smoke.

Dr. Milton examined Tara carefully. Her fever was 101 degrees, and he found swollen lymph glands tucked under the left side of her jaw. "She has an infection in her left ear, Mrs. Smith," Dr. Milton announced after examining both of Tara's ears. "Her eardrum is inflamed and perforated. Have you seen any pus coming out of that ear?"

"No, but she had fever and chills at home. I thought they were a good sign—the body healing itself."

Tara smiled at Dr. Milton. "Daddy gives me medicines to drink and I drink them."

Dr. Milton looked quizzically at Bright Sunshine. "Seneca has studied natural healing. He knows what to do. He's been treating her with herbal teas." Dr. Milton thought she said this with more loyalty than conviction. "But since the ear still hurts, we've come to see you." She paused and added, "Seneca might not approve, but I've come anyway."

Dr. Milton took a bottle of liquid antibiotic from the clinic stock and gave it to Bright Sunshine. He explained to her the importance of using it and the potential dangers of the ear infection. "I know there may be some disagreement in your family about 'Western medicine' but Tara has a serious infection that could get worse. Of course she can keep taking the teas from your husband, but this antibiotic is very important. Very, very important. She must take it, too."

Bright Sunshine agreed to the plan and they departed with Tara waving a chummy good-bye to Dr. Milton.

Somewhat to the surprise of Dr. Milton, Tara returned two days later for the follow-up appointment he had scheduled. This time she was accompanied by her mother and father—a heavy-set man with an unruly blond beard, dirty coveralls, and muddy boots. Tara was much quieter and, Dr. Milton quickly realized, much sicker. Her fever was 103 degrees and she had a piece of tissue wadded in her left ear. "Hi, Dr. Milton," she said. "I don't feel so good." Dr. Milton examined Tara under Seneca's watchful eye. Bright Sunshine sat quietly in the corner of the office. The ear infection was, in fact, much worse, the external ear was tender, the ear canal was filled with pus, and what could be seen of the eardrum was a disturbing scarlet, indicating a raging infection behind it.

"Has she been taking the antibiotic regularly?" Dr. Milton inquired.

"What antibiotic?" barked Seneca.

"The antibiotic I gave Mrs. Smith at the last visit." Seneca looked at Bright Sunshine with a mixture of curiosity and malevolence.

"I knew he wouldn't approve," said Bright Sunshine meekly. "So I told him you said to keep taking the teas—which you did. But we didn't use the bottle of medicine you gave me."

"Antibiotics are body poisons," exclaimed an angry Seneca. "They are anti-natural, a devil's brew. The body needs to heal itself with help from what's in the natural world. Antibiotics don't come from the natural world, they come from techno-capitalism. Our Tara needs to heal herself."

Tara, now a wan, blond child holding her left ear, got off the examination table and climbed onto her mother's lap. Dr. Milton puzzled over what to do next. He discovered that fear was mixed in with his standing concern for Tara. "Mr. and Mrs. Smith, your daughter is very sick. Her ear infection is danger-ous and getting worse. Not only could it damage her hearing permanently, but bone infections, pneumonia, and meningitis are all possibilities. She needs a high dose of medicine that can kill the infection. The only thing we have that can do that is an antibiotic." Dr. Milton emphasized the *we*. Seneca turned a hostile glance from Dr. Milton to Bright Sunshine. "In fact," continued Dr. Milton, "we will need to put her in the hospital so that we can give the medi-cine to her intravenously. This infection is that serious now."

"No way," exploded Seneca. "The hospital is the devil's house. That would damage Tara forever. The body can't possibly heal itself with all the negative energy in a hospital. No damn way she's going to a hospital." Tara and her mother cowered in the corner of the office as Seneca ranted on. "It's the grasses and the seeds and the spores of life that heal mankind. We have an abundance of healing all around us, and you want to put our Tara in a hospital built to make doctors rich and so-called scientists famous? No goddamn way."

Dr. Milton thought of the county Child Protective Services and the police. Would it come to this? In part, though, he was bargaining with the Smiths. He had done this before.

"Mr. and Mrs. Smith. Let me propose this to you. Tara needs medicine now and in high doses. If you will commit—absolutely swear—to give it to her at home, I will wait twenty-four hours before insisting on the hospital. We will give her the first dose here, and you must bring her back to me to check her first thing tomorrow morning." He waited a moment and then added, "I don't want to call in the government protective services folks or get you in trouble with the law, but I'm that worried about your daughter."

Seneca Smith looked compromised and very uncomfortable. He glowered at his wife, "What do you think?"

"I think we'd better do what the doctor says," she responded quickly, hold-ing the feverish Tara tighter.

"OK," said Seneca, "but no needles. You give her the medicine by mouth."

Dr. Milton administered a double dose of the antibiotic to a cooperative Tara under the scowling glare of her father. Dr. Milton reviewed the medication schedule with the Smiths and gave them an appointment for nine o'clock the next morning. Tara waved an enfeebled good-bye to Dr. Milton.

When the Smiths had not arrived by noon the next day, Dr. Milton was very worried. Since they had no phone he decided to spend his lunch hour making a home visit. They lived on the Stowe Mesa, a high flatland east of town transected by multiple arroyos, home to grazing cattle and an occasional ranch house. Dr. Milton pulled down a long, rutted, dirt road to a small, weathered trailer that bore their address. A wood shack—an outhouse—stood to the left of the trailer and a moldering, tireless truck sat in a patch of prairie grass to the right. The door of the trailer was open. "Mr. and Mrs. Smith," he called into the trailer. Silence. "Tara?" A gray cat appeared out of a back room and ambled toward Dr. Milton. He stepped inside and looked around. The three rooms of the trailer were a shambles, all of the shelves bare, the drawers open and empty, and the dirty mattresses shorn of bedding. The kitchen was crusted with dirt, and a badly burned pot sat at the sink. A pile of garbage overwhelmed the small trash can in the corner. In one of the two bedrooms Dr. Milton found a child's drawing taped to the wall, an awkward but accurate portrait of a man with a beard and a woman with a long skirt. Between them was a stick-figure child holding their hands. On a shelf near the picture he found the antibiotic bottle—full.

Dr. Milton drove around the Stowe Mesa trying to find someone who knew the Smiths or where they might have gone. A rancher a mile down the road turned out to be the Smiths' landlord. Not only did he not know that they had departed, he was furious since they owed him rent. He knew nothing about their family or background. He told Dr. Milton that Seneca supported himself doing odd jobs and occasional construction work. No one else seemed to know anything about the Smiths, except that they kept to themselves.

Back in his office, Dr. Milton called Child Protective Services who referred him to the police. He explained what little he knew and that he could not be sure exactly how sick the child was, but that she was definitely in danger. The police assured him that they would distribute some sort of interstate alert and let him know if the Smiths were located.

Dr. Milton went back to work but his spirit was heavy with fear and guilt—fear for Tara and guilt for his own failure to act sooner and harder to protect her. He was comforted a bit by her picture, which he had taken from the trailer and taped to the wall in his office. He consoled himself that many a child had survived purulent ear infections in the days before antibiotics. Surely Tara would too.

Dr. Milton did not see the brief news story that appeared in a Tucson newspaper about a year later. It read as follows:

The State Medical Examiner was called to a remote canyon north of the city to identify human remains that were found yesterday by hunters. The severely desiccated body of a child was located atop a makeshift wooden platform. The medical examiner commented that this form of "burial" was practiced by Indians in some parts of the United States but not this area. Additionally it was reported that the body had blond hair, throwing further doubt on the Indian burial theory. Foul play could not be ruled out. The medical examiner promised further investigation into the case.

Intimate Experiences

In illness, in the permission I as a physician have had to be present at births and deaths, at the tormented battles between daughter and diabolical mother, shattered by a gone brain—just there—for a split second—from one side or the other, it has fluttered before me for a moment, a phrase which I quickly write down on anything at hand, any piece of paper I can grab. It is an indefinable thing, and its characteristic, its chief characteristic is that it is sure, all of a piece and, as I have said, instant and perfect.

—THE AUTOBIOGRAPHY OF WILLIAM CARLOS WILLIAMS

I cannot stay here
to spend my life looking into the past:
the future's no answer. I must
find my meaning and lay it, white,
beside the sliding water: myself—
comb out the language—or succumb

—PATERSON, BOOK 3

The flower dies down
and rots away.
But there is a hole
in the bottom of the bag.

It is the imagination
which cannot be fathomed.
It is through this hole
we escape. . . .

Through this hole
at the bottom of the cavern
of death, the imagination
escapes intact.

—PATERSON, BOOK 5

The Affliction of Flight: A Story

Samuel Shem

For some years I have been afflicted with the belief that flight is possible to man.
—Wilbur Wright

"Aww SHIT! Aw shit!! Aww shit!!!"

Dr. Bill Starbuck had been screaming this intermittently for several days. Occasionally he would sob. It was undignified. It was bestial. It didn't fit with anything anyone knew of the real Bill, long-time doctor for the town, and it was unbearable. Nobody wanted to go into his room.

Before the cursing and sobs had started, Bill had been deteriorating rapidly. At first Orville, his partner and now his doctor, thought that Bill's curses and sobs were signs he might be coming out of his coma. Yet as the minutes and then hours and days wore on, there was no other sign that he was improving. His vital signs were heading in the other direction, showing a failure of many organ systems. Orville's conclusion was that somehow Bill, savvy doctor to the last, was sensing his imminent death and was feeling a lot of pain, in body and soul.

For a while everybody tried harder. Orville increased his attentiveness. Bill's wife Babette intensified her vigil. The nurses worked round the clock to make Bill as comfortable as possible. They even tried squirting hefty doses of his homemade placebo, Starbusol, down the feeding tube, and, at Babette's suggestion—she thinking of the one vegetable he was passionate about—puree of fresh scallions. Nothing made Bill better. He continued his decline.

By now, the ninth of October, the curses and sobs had become fairly continuous. Orville sat at the nursing station, chatting with the nurses and Babette, dreading going into Bill's room for his nightly checkup. Accustomed to dealing with people in pain, Orville knew he wasn't dealing well with this. Lately he had gone to see Bill less and less often, and was now down to the minimum, rounding on him morning and evening. When he was with him, he had been staying for less and less time, doing a brief check of vital signs, a brief physical done with glancing touches, and then leaving, to get away. It was just too much for him to bear. Even Babette, finally, could not sit at his bedside for any length of time, and retreated far down the corridor to the nursing station.

Orville and Babette and the nurses sat there, unable to block out the sobs and the curses. The sounds stirred up images of horror. Much like, Orville thought, Beethoven does, before he lets you off the hook. They tried to get away from the sounds, but the sounds dragged their way down the hallway toward them—like an animal alive in a leg trap. Bill's door had to be shut. Still the sound carried, as if more insistent for its entrapment in the room. Orville heard it as Bill's primal awareness that he would never recover worth shit and that he wished now to die.

Orville realized he couldn't stall any longer. He walked down the hallway toward the hellish sounds, opened the door and went in.

"Aww shit! Aww shit! Aww shit!"

Bill had sunk down on the pillow, as if wanting to burrow under the sheets to go to ground. Only his Humpty Dumpty face was visible. No longer jowly, without those thick glasses, he seemed much younger. His head had edged closer to being a mere skull. The skin seemed to have thinned, veiny and translucent like a baby's, each hill and valley of the bony terrain beneath seeming to shine through, as if lit dimly from within. His thin black hair was mussed, falling forward across his bald top, reminding Orvy of the comic Zero Mostel. Bill's lips were still purled in that girlish way, but more cyanotic. A sign that his heart was less a beat than a whisk, a riff around death.

"Aww shit! Aww shit!"

Bill's eyes were shut. One lowered lid glistened with tears, the other, on the paralyzed side of his face, was dry. Orville thought of his mother, after her brain surgery left her face half-paralyzed, saying, "I *hate* crying out of only one eye!"

He noticed that Bill needed a shave. The nurses had been too broken up lately to do it. When Orville sat down on the bed, Bill started sobbing again. As Orville searched out his carotid for a pulse, Bill barked out: "Aww shit! Aww shit!!

"Aww . . ."

"Stop it, Bill, damn it!" Orville shot back.

Immediately ashamed, he rose and walked to the west-facing window. Terrific. Is that what you've learned this year? To yell at people in pain? The good doctor who can't stand it? Great. Nice work. This contempt is what wrecked your marriage to Lily. This is why you got out of Jersey and ran around the world. He stared out the window. It was dusk. The sun was just down behind the mountains, leaving a fiery red afterglow which was cut sharply by the rise and fall of the frozen pulse of the rock. The river reflected the red as purple, and the purple of the bare-branched orchards and forests as black, the rare lights of the hamlet of Corinth across Middleground Flats, as yellow and red flickers, more like in oil than in water. His town, Columbia, was lighting up against the fall. Its checkerboard—the five long straight streets from river to cemetery and eight cross streets from swamp to swamp, all rotated forty-five degrees off sensible—was pegged by those bold argon streetlights, as if in declaration that any down-and-dirty nightlife would be under the strict illumination of the most high-minded utopians.

He thought of his latest failure in love, Miranda—sad.

A wedge of geese flew past, right to left, heading down river toward Rhinecliff, Poughkeepsie, West Point, Manhattan, past Kill Devil Hill at Kittyhawk and maybe even past Florida toward Columbia's sister city, in Colombia with an *o*, Cartegena. The geese must have been honking as geese normally do, but no sound came through the glass.

When Orville turned back to Bill there was a strong sense that something had changed. It was not definite, and not spooky, yet it called to him clearly. What was it? For some reason he thought of one of his patients, Mrs. Tarr. Several months ago, after her cat Randolph had died, Mrs. Tarr's dry cough worsened. Orville had found lung cancer. She'd never smoked, but sitting in the smoke of the Columbians for forty years in the D.A.R. Library had gotten her. Since diagnosis and treatment, she had gotten rapidly worse. Lately, to him, she was an example of the true-blue Columbians whose blood values and physical state were pretty much incompatible with life. Yet there she was, walking around, alive. Bald from chemo and "into a red turban," toting her mobile oxygen tank to and fro on a leash like she had toted Randolph, sitting in her seat at the borrowing desk at the library, sitting there under the arch of the whale jawbone, checking books in, checking books out. Sometimes even, with Miranda and Amy and Cray and her tank on some Saturdays, still walking the walk in front of the historic Worth Hotel, to try to save it from demolition.

What surprised Orville was the generosity of the Columbians to Mrs. Tarr. People, mostly, had been kind. In tough times, Columbians mostly tried. Helping each other through to the borrowing desk at the library, to the checkout counter at the supermarket, to the parking lot, and, even, beyond. Walking the walk, with oxygen. Coming in the IN door, going out the OUT.

At that moment, turning back to Bill, he saw that his old mentor, here in the best private room in the hospital, had gotten pushed aside, isolated. No one was really with him. He understood, then, what Bill had shown him all those years ago when he'd come to him as a bewildered adolescent, looking for somebody with some sense—no, more, with some *expanse*. Bill hadn't told him, no. He had shown him. Through his being with patients and laying on his hands and saying "heh heh" and taking a crate of scallions or a chicken as payment, Bill had shown him that what healed people had less to do with diagnosing and treating, and more to do with connecting.

For the first time Orville understood the force of isolation. Even in the face of cancer, or coma. Understood, also, that the moments of healing were when he had, often inadvertently, been present with people. Bill had shown him that this is what good doctors do to heal. We're present at the crucial moments, he said to himself, and in the ordinary moments. We bring someone who is out on the edge of the so-called sick into the current of the human. We take what seems foreign in a person, and see it as native. This is healing. This is what good doctors do. Isolation is deadly. Connection heals. Even in dying.

What Orville understood then about Bill was that this dear old doc who'd been in the thick of connection with the town for much of a century was now totally isolated. If he were to stay in this room with him, he had to be with him.

Yeah, Mr. Big Shot Doctor, he said to himself, and how do you do that, eh?

Mundanely. Down to earth. Don't be a hero. Do something small.

Dr. Rose decided to give Dr. Starbuck a shave. After all, the first doctors, the surgeons, had evolved from barbers, had they not?

Orville's constant transitions from finishing his day or night as a doctor and starting his night or day as a person had taught him to carry, in his black bag, a shaving kit. He took out his wooden shaving mug and a safety razor and screwed together the chrome-plated Crabtree and Evelyn genuine badger-bristle shaving brush. He filled a bowl with steaming hot water and worked it into a lather. As he propped Bill up higher, the slippage of the sheets down from his neck was like an exhumation. The scent was that terrible mix of stale sweat and residual excrement and urine and baby powder that was too familiar to doctors and nurses, signifying bodily decay and hospital neglect.

How light Bill's head is! he thought. As if he's not walking these last steps, but flying them.

He began to lather Bill's face. It wasn't easy to shave someone else. The brush felt awkward on Bill's skin. Try to feel his face from *his* side. What if you could do that anytime you chose? Shift from "I" to "you," take on the other as self? Better yet, take on all of it—"I" and "you" and "we"? What if you could go through a day without using the word "I"?

As he worked the brush, trying to feel it working from Bill's side, chin-to-sideburn, cheek-to-fallen-lip-corner, it started to feel different. As if he were working it on his own face, in that unconscious way you get into, so habitually that if you try to do it you can't do it at all. And then he began to sense it as if he were working it up and down and back and forth across the face of the town.

Bill continued to curse and weep. When Orville started floating the razor through the lather he had to time his strokes carefully. He set to work.

"Oh you shouldn't have to do that, Dr. Rose." A nurse in the doorway. She was tall and of Columbian weight. A moon face and slight moustache and hirsutism and widow's hump to her neck. Diagnosis? Incipient Cushing's syndrome, a disorder of the adrenals.

"No, that's okay," he said. "I'll finish him up."

"But it's not your job," she said. "I'll call a Candy-Striper."

"I want to do it."

"But it's against regulations."

Orville started to see red. He was about to lash out at her. But then he saw her not only as she was but as her story, her life. He knew it well, for she had been a classmate of his in high school, and a patient of Bill's and his. He saw her as the farmer's daughter who'd gotten involved with one of the brutes who impregnated her in her junior year, so she dropped out in disgrace and had twin girls, and the brute, when they were about one year old, was finishing up bathing one girl and came out and the other had fallen into the diaper pail and drowned. Things went to hell. The brute left. Single motherhood. Somehow pulled herself up and became a nurse, a stickler for regulations but a good nurse. You don't recover from that, Orville said to himself, from that baby in the diaper pail; you don't recover, you change. And she had. His heart softened.

"I'm sorry, Cindy," he said, softly. He was saying that he was sorry for her tragedy and appreciating her making it, at least, into nursing and into this room with Bill and him and the falling away. "I want to do something for Bill, some last thing, before he dies."

His softening softened her. Tears came to her eyes. "Sorry, Orvy," she said. "You go ahead. Call when . . .if you need us?"

"I will."

She left. He resumed shaving.

With Bill's sobbing and cursing it wasn't a neat job. Nicks oozed poorly oxygenated blood the color of a sluggish stream at dusk. He stopped the oozing with a styptic pencil. As Orville got into it, feeling, as a guide through the lather under his fingertips, Bill's bristly skin, it was as if he were feeling his own stubble, and the razor cutting through his own lather. And then, under his attention it transformed again, so it wasn't even that he was shaving Bill or shaving himself, but that shaving was happening. So, he thought, either there is attention or there is "me"—take your pick. The shaving became a suturing up, across a mirror, across a fleshy gap.

He wiped the last flecks of lather away, and took out his bottle of Aloe Vera with Swiss Herbs hand creme that he used to keep the skin of his too-often-washed hands from cracking and splitting. He massaged it into Bill's papery skin, softening it. When he finished it seemed almost lambent.

"Okay, Bill," he said, "now you get the extra-special, super-duper treatment, for only our best customers. Miranda gave me this." He took out a spritzer of Caswell-Massey Cologne Spray Number 6, which she told him was the one made by the same firm two hundred years ago for the Father of Our Country, George Washington. It wasn't until he'd George Washington'd Bill up that he realized the old guy had fallen silent.

Orville was startled.

Something else is happening. In him, in me, in us, beyond us. I'm his mother now, he's my son. Help him go.

Fear came over him, fear of failing Bill and fear of being seen doing what he was about to do, something others would take to be really abnormal.

He pumped the bottle of skin creme and took Bill's hand and stroked it firmly with the goo, drawing the skin over the bones so that he was making deep contact, the knuckles like marbles in a child's velvet bag, the bones like long stones. He bent to Bill's ear.

"You can go now, Bill."

Orville's only clue to his getting through to him as he moved on to his chest, the ribbed box above his thrumming bird's heart, was his own feeling inside his own chest, an answering thrum, a chill, a sense of excitement and sadness all at once at a leaving and also an arrival. Bill is leaving and arriving, he thought, and I am arriving and leaving, and it's the same trip really.

Bill was still. Breathing lightly but still. Announcing that he was now dying. His dying is forcing me to announce that I'm still living, right here, right now with this old man. It isn't his heart or my heart, it's the human heart, the human journey, common and ordinary, and a big deal and a small deal both, and the only deal really and available to us all at no extra cost if we can face it, bear it, share it.

The moment wasn't mystical or sad or scary or corny, it was just a moment. It shone.

Having forgotten to spray Bill's thorax with George Washington, Orville went back and did it, whispering in Bill's ear, "Hey old friend, you can go now, you see?"

And so on down his body, patting his still-fat tummy, this little boy's universal tummy that a mother had once patted with such delight, white as that of a fish and scaled with gray curly hairs whorled like galaxies, patting it playfully patty-cake, patty-cake.

"You're going out a little under your fighting weight, Bill, but it's okay."

And even Bill's groin, the shrunken purple-tipped penis that may have had its share of adventures in repayment for his tending the whores on Diamond Street.

"Two dollars a house call," Bill had told him, "and I never came away empty-handed, heh heh."

"Hey you old rogue," Orvy whispered, "you had some great times, and you can go now, too." And those shriveled plums that had kept churning out those whippy-tailed big-headed sperm, like factories in a war effort and which, because of the deadly PCBs in the Hudson River or the cement dust in the air, had fertilized Babette's eggs to produce two neurological disasters for children, the boy dead, the girl wheelchaired—all of this Orville moistened and spritzed with cologne and talked to. He took out his comb and combed Bill's thin hair.

"You can go now, Bill."

Orville was finished. He arranged Bill's flaccid gleaming limbs in as dignified a position as possible and drew the sheet back up, leaving the arms and hands outside, palms up, reminding him of the Buddha and of Celestina Polo in that hotel room in Largo del'Orta, Italy. Sitting there still for a moment, in silence, Orville knew that he was talking not just to Bill, but to his mother as well. She was still dead and had stopped flying around. He felt a rush, a many-colored yearning, rocking him back in his chair. He tried to get his arms around what he yearned for. It was the same heartrending yearning he'd felt for the woman he loved when he lost her, and for the little boy. Maybe the yearning is feeling seen by death, a boy gone.

He walked to the door and gestured down the hallway for the nurse. He asked her to bring in Babette.

Babette came quickly. She had changed into a billowing muumuu with hibisci in bloom and a panther about to pounce, and a straw hat sporting guavas ringed with bananas. She saw, in his glance, what was what.

"No, not yet!" she cried out. "Please no."

Orville brought her to Bill's bedside. She removed her hat.

"He looks so sweet," she blurted out. Tears were running through her makeup like rain through dust. "So young. He's like a little baby: Sweet. And he smells so nice."

Orville took her hand and showed her how to massage his hand, his cheek, with him. Soon her hand relaxed. He felt her feeling what he had felt: her husband's torment had lessened, lightened. As if the light from the room had been drawn into him. Within that body lying there. Almost a glow.

She started sobbing. Orville put his arm around her broad back. She cried into his neck. The spasm left. She pulled away.

"Babette," he said, "listen." He turned to Bill, and put his hand upon his open palm and said firmly, "You can go now, Bill."

"No! No you can't!" She tugged Orville's hand away and held it up above the sheets.

"Go on." He put her hand once again on Bill's open palm. "You tell him." They sat motionless, and silent, for what seemed a long time.

Babette moved Bill's hand, in hers, to her lap. Looking down at it shyly like a little girl who is talking to an imaginary friend so important that she's more real than a live one, she asked, "Scally?"

Embarrassed, she looked up at Orville and said, "That's what I called him, y'know, all these years, our secret name. 'Scally' for the scallions he loved so much? He called me that name too, 'Scally.' We never told anybody, it was so silly—'Dr. and Mrs. Scally,' we called ourselves and we laughed—oh, we laughed. It was silly but it was ours, our whole lives . . ."

She broke down again. Then, lifting her head to look at Bill squarely, and with each word more sure, she became the wife, the woman who had stayed right there with him just like this all these years, no matter what. The woman who had, in a pinch, shown up with him and helped him as a good mother might. Through the illness and death of their second child and the illness and decay of their first, through the trials of doctoring Columbians and through all the secrets and truth of the life of the town that they shared, because the only person he could tell them to was her.

"Scally, did you hear me? It's all right. You . . . you . . ." She turned to Orvy. "I can't!" He smiled at her. Put a hand on her shoulder.

"You . . . you can go now, my . . . my dearest love."

They both felt a wave of sorrow. Tears came to Orville's eyes, eased down his cheeks. Babette sobbed hard. Her whole body shook. The plastic banana earrings swung wildly against her neck, trees in a hurricane.

They sat together on Bill's bed. Everything was still.

As they calmed they became aware that the light had gone out of Bill. His spirit was gone. Orville leaned over and felt for a carotid pulse. Still there, some. His body was not dead, but his spirit was somewhere else. You could never have measured it, yet for the past hour Orville had felt it had been there, as the pilot flame of a furnace in an old house is there—and now it was not. There, not.

Babette wept more gently now, tears of release washing out the fear.

"He'll be all right now, dear," Orville said, rising. His hand still rested on her shoulder, much as Bill's, at the right times, had rested on his. "He'll be fine."

A few nurses were in the doorway.

"He'll be going now," he said, "soon."

They began to cry. He started to make his way out, past them, feeling really old. Old age suddenly spread its wings in him, and he felt the creaking of betrayal.

"Are you leaving?" Babette cried out, again fearful.

"No, dear. I'll just be down the hall at the nursing station."

Bill's body kept on for a few more hours of its eighty-third year in the world and then stopped. By that time, their tears had softened, washed of fear. What was there to be afraid of anymore? The softened tears were those of surrender to Bill's life, to the way his life had been aligned with all of theirs for both a long time and a brief time and a final time. The surrender was to being part of something else, which can't help but bring a sense of awe.

Like, Orville thought, when you stand in a redwood grove and look up or stand on a canyon rim and look down or—my dream!—hold a baby in your arms who one day, if you're lucky, will be holding you in his arms, and you realize that your life is a speck in the time of that redwood or the dirt of that canyon or the revolution of that baby and that man. The awe of being a part of the whole, even for a moment of your life.

Suddenly out of nowhere came a crush of despair, knocking him down, mercilessly down. Stunned. Desperate.

I'm alone! Alone! Who can I call? Miranda? No. Who?

He looked at the clock. Past midnight. Morning in Rome. He picked up the phone.

Mr. Tron's Farewell

Elissa Ely

IN THE COURSE of human events, pregnancies occur. But when you are a pregnant doctor in the hospital, there aren't many honest reasons for anyone else to celebrate. For other doctors, it means maternity leave: months of stretched and stressful coverage. For patients, it simply means abandonment. From that time onward, even after you return, deflated and unslept, you stand transparently with one foot in that other world—that involving, distracting, revealed place where you mostly live now, with children who, by the laws of nature, matter more than anything else. Patients are encouraged to depend on doctors, who then abandon them. It's psychiatrically messy.

I had been pregnant for several months. I had not disclosed it yet. I was feeling like one of those squat, abdominally obstructive Mafioso kings who must be helped up by his associates after polishing off a platter of lasagna in the back room of a cappuccino joint where a mob hit has just been committed. I was short-tempered, over-stuffed, and not able to hide the condition any longer.

The patients noticed it first. One morning, a small astute woman with worries came up to me on the unit and stared. "Dr. Ely," she said, "you look big. Are you pregnant?"

"I am," I said, relieved someone had finally come out with it.

"Oh," she said, and thought a minute. "Am I?" she asked.

After that, there were no more secrets. Medical staff swore they had known for weeks, but hadn't wanted to be first to mention it. Patients were immediately involved.

"I hate you, I hate you!" a woman screamed down the corridor after we revoked her privileges. "I can't stand the ground you walk on . . . and *Congratulations On Your Baby!*"

A man with few intelligible words sidled up. Most of the time, he was lost at war, preoccupied with artillery and sick count.

"When you gonna stop being so fat?" he said.

"I'll stop being so fat when the baby comes."

"You having a baby?"

"That's right."

"Well," he said, "then you better take off a shoe and drink some hot chocolate."

These were patients who would survive separation. Their solicitudes were diffuse, their curiosity general. There was another patient whose survival was less clear. Growing up in Vietnam, he had wanted to be a doctor. On a tiny boat to America, his family was murdered by pirates. He learned English in California, and worked as a painter when he could. Employment was fitful, and he grew angry. His thoughts began to fly. They took on a speed of their own. He started to hear Voices. The Voices convinced him to set a house on fire. It burned to the ground. The Voices convinced him several more times before he was caught.

Most delusions step no farther than the edge of the self: dark forces are after you and only you, or special powers make you and only you extraordinary. His arsons were altruistic. In his speeding mind, he believed that a series of successful fires would enrich employment opportunities for immigrant carpenters, men like himself who searched honestly but could find no jobs. His purpose was to create a market.

We met in the hospital. He was sleepless with mania and wild with pain from a mouthful of dangling teeth. Nerves were rotting but he refused all help, bellowing in broken English and threatening to kill anyone who approached. His quiet wife brought him rice and his sons hung fearfully in the visitor's hallway.

He was forced to take medication. I signed the order for the first dose, and while the nurse drew it up, male staff pulled on plastic gloves. Hip exposed to the needle, he looked up at me in the doorway and swore revenge. Over the next weeks, the medication began to help. First, he slept. Then, he stopped bellowing. Then, he saw the hospital dentist, lost some of his teeth and took antibiotics for the rest. He ate hospital food and put on weight. His new self met me without his old self's vengeance. He talked about going home. He wanted to support his wife. He did not want the money of the state. He never talked about the voices or the fires. In his right mind, shame was clear but silent.

The community refused to take him back. He had created too many memories. An arsonist has no second life. Even compensated, he was too dangerous for discharge. They resisted for several years, while various consultants on either side wrote authoritative opinions. The chart grew thick. He took his medications, worked in the hospital canteen, looked through the employment ads in the paper, went quietly home on weekends.

Finally, forced by his progress, the community agreed to accept him on one condition: that he continue to meet with me. It was an unorthodox arrangement. Our meetings appeared to be for his medications, but were in fact so that someone else could worry about him regularly.

My office was just outside the Unit doors. When he returned each week, he never looked through the window onto the floor where he had lived, but would hurry off the elevator into the room, and hurry out of the room onto the elevator. He was always on time, though the trip was long and he had no car. Our visits interrupted his search for work, and, when he found a house-painting job, our visits interrupted his schedule. But he came steadily.

He had become a quiet man, and we were an old couple by now: conversation was abbreviated and referential. While I wrote out prescriptions, he spoke shyly about his cooking (he had taken up cooking now that he could chew), and his boys, who had American nicknames and played videogames. We did not talk about his life in Vietnam. We did not talk about his illness. We certainly did not talk about his plans for the future. Constancy and compliance were what the community required of him. They wanted weekly proof of his sanity.

We met in this mild forum for years. But pregnancy was going to put an end to it. He was too delicate and controversial a patient to hand over to a substitute. It was destabilizing to switch his care once and then switch back again. The community had found a clinic for him at last. His case would be transferred.

He said nothing when I told him we would have to say goodbye before the baby was born. He had lost family, country, and sanity. Then he smiled. His teeth were yellow and in need of care, but routinely so.

"A baby!" he said. "Alright! No sleep for Doctah!" He leaned forward and pumped my hand. He spoke a little too fast and too loud. I made a worried note.

He was late for our last meeting. I was tamping down the loose administrative ends of coverage, too tired in the ninth month to care about transferential meanings or the pertinent feelings about farewell. Those are subtle discussions, and I was too large for subtlety. I was the right size only for annoyance. If not showing was how he wished to say goodbye, then, goodbye. It was a traditional but unimaginative way to give the doctor the raspberry.

The old elevator, never in much of a hurry itself, creaked up to the floor. I heard it stop. When the door opened, a dozen roses stepped off. There was a cake behind them, and a number of people behind the cake. An off-key tenor was singing vigorously without any R's. "You ahhh so beautiful to me," the voice sang. He had brought his family. The boys with American nicknames kicked the walls and his wife smiled timidly. They looked uncomfortable. He looked delighted.

We ate the cake, which he zestfully served piece by piece. He was talking fast; the words were starting to speed. He noted, almost gaily and in passing, that in his country his large family had eaten a single meal a day. There had never been parties with cakes. He stood and sat and stood and produced a box with wild ribbons and holographic wrap. A blanket for a giant's child fell out. Then he brought out a camera he had borrowed, and his wife took a picture, the kind that floats up before your eyes into figures. We looked at it. One of us was all tooth, the other all stomach. "You ah so beautiful," he said, laughing loudly, "and I am so ugly."

The gay moment was filled with loss. It called for anger and sadness. This brightness was all wrong. People come apart from farewells. I smelled flames around the edge of the room, and wondered who else ought to know he was burning.

"Goodbye now, Doctor, I so happy for you," he shouted, shaking my hand, and then he ducked out of the office. His sons ducked out after him. I could hear them all poking the down button riotously. His wife lingered. She was timid, but had something to say.

"When he heard you was having a baby," she said, making careful words, "he come home and said that same thing to me: 'I so happy.' 'Why you happy?' I asked him. 'Now you won't see doctor anymore! You lose! Why be happy about that?'"

It was my fear exactly.

"He said to me, 'I happy because now doctor never be lonely again.' He worried for you loneliness."

When a dangerous person has everything to lose, it is training to think diagnostically. A loud laugh and rambling thoughts are the first noises of mania. Generosity at those moments is so rare it is hardly recognizable. Generosity at those moments is something between an embrace and a collapse, a way of holding off the flames, and very brave.

"That how he is, you know," his wife said.

The Ballad of the Bird Lady

MAUREEN RAPPAPORT

WORDS ARE BEAUTIFUL, standing alone on a white sheet, or gliding through the air. If my first love were letters, my second would be numbers, and throughout my daily rounds of tending to the sick I call upon the power of both to help me.

It is natural to grow attached to a patient after weeks, and months, and years of visits, and since a large part of my practice includes geriatrics, death seems to be lurking behind many doors. Watching life sift through my fingers like sand would be unbearable were it not for the ink that gathers and shapes it into a perfect circle of story.

Mrs. G. had been mostly healthy in the seven years I have known her. By the age of eighty, most people have stopped pretending to be what they are not and have assumed truly unique personalities. Mrs. G. was no exception. She loved to talk, and being a childless widow, with only a canary as a companion, her visits to the doctor were more of a social affair than a medical one. I enjoyed these visits as much as she did, but it was inevitable that one day disease would come between us.

Last year, at the age of eighty-six, Mrs. G. developed a pain in her belly which didn't respond to her usual cure of dandelion stems. I sent her for a barium enema, which showed an apple-core lesion in her ascending colon. This meant cancer.

"Why don't they just leave us old people alone?" she said when I told her the bad news. I wasn't sure if she was referring to the deities responsible for dishing out her disease or the doctors (myself included) for suggesting nasty treatments!

Not knowing what else to do after referring her to a specialist, I offered to take care of her bird, Joey, during her hospitalization for surgery.

My kids liked Joey, though he was old and scraggly like his owner. Half his feathers were missing. Tamara, my little daughter, thought he must be too sad and worried over the little-old lady to sing. I brought my children with me to Mrs. G's apartment when she was strong enough to take her bird back.

"She's really old," whispered Tammy from behind my legs as she peeked at the bird lady.

Mrs. G. has been in and out of the hospital this past year and should have gone to a hospice for terminal care but preferred to go back to her own apartment with help from a visiting nurse and homemaker. Notified of the arrangements, I was happy to resume her medical care as part of the home-care team.

Remembering the time I visited her with my kids, I wondered what had become of the old bird as I made my way up to her apartment.

Mrs. G. kept the chain on her door as she wedged her face in the crack to see who was there. She was expecting me.

"You look like you lost weight," she said.

The skin drawn over her face, exposing bones I never saw before, shocked me. I almost responded, "Look who's talking." Instead I smiled and waited politely as she inched her way with a walker to an armchair in the living room.

"I'm slow, you pass me and sit on the couch," she commanded.

It was a mystery to me how she managed alone. Her legs were grotesquely deformed; lymphedema and peau d'orange are the proper medical terms for a leg swollen to six times its usual size, encased in shiny, bluish-red skin. She must have weighed only fifty pounds, her legs accounting for at least twenty of those pounds.

"Joey must have heard you," she mused as she stopped to catch her breath before finally plopping down in her chair.

I looked into her kitchen surprised to find the old, yellow canary pecking at his cage, looking as fit as ever.

"And how are the children?" Mrs. G. asked.

We talked about my children, about the value of fresh calf's liver, about her neighbors. She talked about the same things during each of my weekly visits but never complained of pain or hardship.

Last week Mrs. G. began vomiting. Her belly hardened all over, and the lump in her right lower quadrant pushed out like a baby's head at forty weeks. Her nephew found her lying on the floor. She could no longer manage alone.

This morning I visited her in the hospital. I found her curled up, like a little bird, on a bed on Five Main, dying.

"Who's going to take care of Joey?" I asked, when I really wanted to ask if she knew she was dying. While still at home, Mrs. G. spoke as if her swollen legs and the lump in her belly would get better.

"I guess it's time for him to die," she said.

I couldn't stop the tears from falling down my cheeks as I told her I had written a story about her and her bird.

She smiled—a real smile. Church bells began chiming as she continued to smile. She stopped blinking; her pupils remained dilated. For one horrible instant I thought she was on her way to heaven and, despite all my experience, I was afraid! But as I looked down at her bony chest, I saw it rise and fall, her breath trembling.

And I trembled, too.

The Fascination of What Is Difficult

John Lantos

For Rebecca, the best thing about Pittsburgh was the view as she emerged from the Fort Pitt tunnel on sunny mornings. The three rivers, the fountain at the point, the boats, the stadium, the funky architecture of the corporate skyscrapers crowded into the triangle of downtown always got her dreaming of river trips down the Ohio and the Mississippi, into New Orleans, and on to the Gulf. In other ways, the move to Pittsburgh from New York had been pretty depressing. She could get good bagels in Squirrel Hill, but there was a sense of being closed in, a sense that what happened in Pittsburgh didn't really matter. She felt that she was just doing time there.

She also knew that, as a philosopher, she should be happy just having a job, and that her job teaching medical ethics was a plum. No more explaining Hume and Kant to bored undergraduates fulfilling distribution requirements. She could move beyond theory, make a difference in people's lives. It was heady, life and death stuff. The students, hobbled as they were by the premed curriculum, the brutal medical school selection process, and the mindless reductionism of medical education, didn't get half of what she was trying to teach them, but some of them seemed interested and appreciative. There were the others, too, of course, the ones who would say, "Just tell us what to do not to get sued."

Today, she was meeting for the first time the third-year students on pediatrics. Bob Schmidt, a pediatrician who'd been teaching ethics before she arrived, had called and asked her to work with him. He had a reputation as the best teacher around. He told her that he didn't know much about ethics, but hoped they could work together, since he thought it was important.

"What should we teach them?" he asked.

"We could do neonates, Baby Doe stuff," she suggested.

"I hate neonatology."

She smiled. She did too.

"What about something to do with transplants?" This was Pittsburgh, after all. "We could do a case where there is one liver, two patients. Talk about resource allocation, tragic choices, all that stuff."

"I never talk to the third years about liver transplants. They're here to learn how to be doctors, not how to provide spare parts."

Was this guy for real?

"Well, what do you want to talk about?"

"Why don't we do something simple? Truth-telling. How do you tell somebody that their child has a terrible disease. Do you ever do role-plays?"

"I could."

"OK, here's what we'll do. You be the doctor. I'll be the parent of a kid who has just been diagnosed with a brain tumor. You have to tell me my kid has cancer and that he's going to die."

"Sounds good. Should I do a little introductory talk about the moral basis of truth-telling?"

"If you want."

She looked forward to meeting him.

She parked in her own, private parking space. She'd negotiated hard for that.

When she walked past the ER, she thought of the time she'd taken her daughter in. The doctors had been worried about meningitis. They did a spinal tap, blood tests, X-rays, kept Liana in for three days on IV antibiotics. It turned out to be a virus or something. Whenever doctors don't know what's going on, they say it's a virus. She had not been a very good parent, didn't listen to anything the doctor said, bugged the nurses, cried all night. The residents had a nickname for people like her, WAPs, White Anxious Parents.

She followed the blue painted lines to the Little Mermaid elevators and went up to the Ronald McDonald conference room on the eighth floor. There were ten or twelve students there already. Dr. Schmidt hadn't arrived yet. The students were wearing the short white coats that, as she'd learned, symbolized inexperience. Some had rubber tourniquets tied to their buttonholes, bulky stethoscopes around their necks, and their pockets were bulging with Harriet Lane Handbooks and other doctor self-help books. A couple of the women had little furry panda bears clasping their stethoscopes. Rebecca thought how vulnerable and impressionable the students looked. She liked opening their minds to the world beyond the medical sciences. She passed around a recent article from the *New England Journal* showing that doctors frequently lied to their patients.

The door opened and Dr. Schmidt walked in, chattering away, "Lisa, what happened to that kid with the cellulitis?"

"It grew strep pneumo."

"What's he on?"

"We changed him from cefuroxime to ampicillin. His temp is down. He looks better."

"Good, good. Barry, what about your baby with RSV?"

"They still didn't give him the ribavirin."

"Those damn ICU docs don't know a virus from an ET tube. Just 'cause they can put in big lines, they think they can do anything. Is he getting better?

"A little."

"What else is going on?"

"We got a new HIV kid."

"Oh shit. Who picked him up?"

"I did."

"Derrick, Derrick, just 'cause you're black, doesn't mean you have to be Albert Schwitzer. Let somebody else have a tragedy once in while. The honkeys gotta learn this stuff sometime."

The black guy smiled. Rebecca couldn't believe it. She'd been in the medical school for a year and had never met an attending physician who knew the medical students' names, knew who was following which patients, and could acknowledge the fact that not everyone was white. And she had seldom seen students respond to an attending physician with anything but boredom, deference, or fear. This guy acted like he was their friend, and they acted like they wanted to be his. She was intrigued. She wanted to impress him.

"Hi," she said, "I'm Rebecca."

He smiled, held out his hand, didn't quite meet her eye.

"Nice to meet you."

He had a bushy, blondish-gray beard. He was overweight. He was wearing a polo shirt, chinos, clogs. She'd heard somewhere that his parents were missionaries, that he'd grown up traveling from one emerging African country to another. She'd heard about a recent, messy divorce. She wondered if he was seeing anyone. Didn't look like it.

"You have a little talk ready?" he asked.

She nodded.

"OK, boys and girls, pay attention," he sounded almost schoolmarmish, maybe just the slightest bit sarcastic. "We're going to talk about ethics here. Philosophy is much more important to practicing medicine than histology, so no dozing. Put down those newspapers and listen."

She turned on the slide projector and started in. She dramatically recounted the story of the Tuskegee syphilis study, how hundreds of rural black men had been studied by the U.S. Public Health Service for years without being told they had syphilis or that a treatment was available. She summarized the legal cases that first codified the doctrine of informed consent. She alluded to Kant, the categorical imperative, the principle of patient autonomy, and the need to respect people as individuals, even if they disagree with us. She brought in some psychological theory, transference and countertransference, how doctors are sometimes afraid of death and project those fears onto the patient, but how studies showed that patients, even children, were much better able to deal with dismal information than doctors thought. She talked about changes in clinical practice, which gave many patients real choices among different treatments, such as lumpectomy or mastectomy for breast cancer. She showed how all these strains of modern thought, philosophy, law, psychology, and clinical epidemiology converged to form a moral obligation to tell patients the truth, even though it was sometimes difficult. And she did it all in fifteen minutes. She felt good about herself. This was what she did best. Schmidt applauded, the students joined in tentatively, and he then told them to take a five-minute break.

While they were out of the room, he sat down beside Rebecca. "OK," he said, "here's the situation. I'm from southern West Virginia. I just brought my kid in because he had a seizure. After the seizure, he couldn't speak. They transferred him up here to see a neurologist. You just got the MRI results that show an inoperable brain tumor. The chest X-ray shows mets to the lungs. He is going to die. I'm his dad. You're going to tell me the bad news."

"Got it." She was a little nervous. Giving a talk was one thing. She knew what she was going to say. This was a whole different sort of performance.

The students filed back in with bags of chips, cups of coffee. The room was warm. Rebecca noticed the anatomic diagrams on the wall showing the nerves to the leg and the arm. She thought about those different images of the body, how medicine allowed us to know things about other people that had never been knowable before. She remembered those ads in comic books for X-ray glasses. You could look at clothed people and see them naked! Outside the window, she could see the gothic spires of the Cathedral of Learning.

Schmidt announced that they were going to do a little role-play, and asked the students to decide what they were doing that was right or wrong. He nodded to Rebecca, then sat down in a chair by the window, his head down. He seemed to be meditating. Or dozing. The students settled down.

She borrowed a white coat from one of the medical students and liked the way it felt. She took the stethoscope out of the pocket and slung it around her neck. She walked over to Schmidt and sat down beside him. He was looking at the floor and didn't look up. She was aware of being watched, of being judged. She put her hand lightly on his knee. He jumped.

"Mr. Schmidt?"

"Yeah?"

"Hi. I'm Dr. Goldberg. One of the pediatricians."

"Oh, hi Doctor." He jumped up, grabbed her hand, started pumping it.

"It's nice to meet you." He got the Appalachian twang down just about right. "Mah doctor down in Meadow Bridge said y'all up here in Pittsburgh would be able to help my boy. I didn't wanna go so far, didn't seem that serious but he insisted, so here I am. I sure am glad to meet y'all. This is quite a hospital. Never seen anything so big."

He really gets into this, she thought. She started to get into it, too. And it suddenly seemed a little harder than she expected.

"Mr. Schmidt. I need to tell you what we've found out about your son."

"Dwight," he said, "he's my only boy. Had four girls, then Dwight. Thought I'd never get a boy, but I told my wife, bless her heart, that we had to jus' keep on trying. He's a holy terror, too. Let me tell you. Whups those girls good. We went huntin' together last year. He got a deer his first day out. Eight years old! This year, I'm gonna surprise him at Christmas time and get him his own gun."

"What I wanted to tell you, Mr. Schmidt, is that we've done some, ah, tests, on your boy, your son, on, I mean, Dwight, and ah, we think we have the diagnosis."

"Goddamn," he chuckled, "I knew you guys were good. Dr. Ushan, back home, she's all right. I mean, her English ain't so good but she seems to know what she's doing with colds and stuff, but once he had this seizure, well, she knew she was in over her head. And hey, I've heard about those transplants y'all do up here, livers, hearts, guts, everything, stem to stern. I'll bet you'll be doin' brain transplants pretty soon, people need 'em. So, how long'll Dwight have to be in. We gotta get back and do some hayin'."

"Well, Mr. Schmidt, the tests show that he has a brain tumor."

"A what?"

"A tumor."

He stared at her, looking blank, puzzled.

"What do you mean?"

"Well, it's a growth, something growing, and we think it might be cancer." She couldn't believe her own words. She knew it was cancer, but even in a role-play, even though she was just pretending, it was hard to say the word. Schmidt looked at her. She thought she saw him wink. Just for a second, she was really angry with him. She turned away, took a breath, noticed the students. They were leaning forward. No papers were rustling. Nobody was looking at their books or out the window, the way they were during her lecture. She could imagine their eager criticism of her evasions. She turned back to Schmidt, pitiless.

"Mr. Schmidt, I'm very sorry to tell you this, but your son has brain cancer," she said; "He's going to die."

"Cancer? He had a seizure. They said he had a seizure."

"Sometimes cancer causes seizures."

"Cancer causes seizures?"

"It can. If it's brain cancer."

"Well, what can we . . . I mean, what are you going to do? How long will he have to be in?"

"Mr. Schmidt, let's sit down?"

"No ma'am, I'm fine here. I'm just fine here. I just want to know how long it'll take to get rid of it, I mean till he'll be OK."

"Mr. Schmidt, I told you, your son is going to die. The cancer has spread to his lungs. There's nothing we can do. I'm very sorry." She wondered if she was really doing this right. He seemed to be making it as hard for her as he could. She felt like he despised her.

Schmidt walked over to the window. He looked out for a few moments. She wasn't sure whether the role-play was over. Suddenly, he turned back to face her. He looked enraged. He walked slowly over and stuck a finger in her face. She was afraid he was going to hit her. She'd had enough of this. She was ready to quit.

"Look, what're you, a nurse? Can I see a real doctor?"

Blood rushed to her face.

"Mr. Schmidt, Mr. Schmidt . . ."

"I want to talk to a doctor, not some dipshit nurse. I want to talk to someone around here who is not so fucking stupid that they can't take care of a kid with a seizure. Don't you tell me my son is going to die. You don't know shit. He ain't going to die. We're going hunting this fall."

He stormed out of the room. She was glad to see him go. She wasn't going to teach with him anymore. This wasn't medical ethics; this was some asshole using her and the students for his own weird catharsis. Clearly, he had just wanted to embarrass her in front of the students. She looked at them. A couple of them were sniffling. Nobody met her eyes.

Schmidt walked slowly back into the room, transformed once again into a chubby pediatrician. He came over, gave her a hug, and said, "Nice job. Best performance I've seen. From a philosopher." He smiled. She couldn't meet his eyes.

"You OK?" he asked.

Did she smell alcohol on his breath? Something was wrong with this guy. She wasn't sure if she loved him or hated him, whether she should try to help him or report him to someone. He turned to the students and said, "How'd she do?"

"I thought she did really well, but she, at first, she didn't really tell the truth about the cancer."

"Was that a problem?"

"Well, everybody says you should tell patients the truth. Informed consent and all that?"

"Why didn't you tell the truth, at first?" Schmidt asked.

"I don't know. You seemed so unprepared to hear it. It seemed like maybe the best thing to do would be to ease into it, give you a little bit at the first meeting and a little more later on."

"Yes!" Schmidt nearly shouted. "That may be right." He paused. "You know, everybody says 'Tell the truth, tell the truth,' as if that's an easy thing to do. It's easy to say. But hard to do. The hard thing is knowing when to lie. Telling the truth can be an awful thing. Sometimes, you just can't do it. And sometimes, maybe you shouldn't, though I'm not sure exactly when. I don't always do it. And sometimes, it's the hardest thing you will ever have to do. Much harder than transplanting a liver. What were y'all feeling during the scene?"

"Man, it seemed like you just hated her," Derrick said. "I felt bad for her. You were givin' her a pretty hard time."

"Yeah, well, you're going to get that. But just remember that they're not really mad at you. As a doctor, you represent not just healing but also disease. Those twin snakes! You sometimes hold the power to cure. But you also have terrible knowledge, bring terrible news, and it's a lot harder for people to get mad at the news than to get mad at you. Part of the reason why it's so hard to tell the truth: It hurts."

He turned to leave, turned back.

"Work rounds tomorrow at eight. We'll meet on the eighth floor. Who's on tonight?"

Two students raised their hands.

"Call me if you have any questions. I like to be called. I get lonely at home."

He left. The students filed slowly out.

Rebecca wondered what truths he had not told.

Into the Light

WILLIAM J. POMIDOR

"DID YOU HEAR about the eclipse?" Elizabeth asks. She glances at me over the top of her surgical mask, her thick eyebrows fluttering question marks. Between us is an incubator, a clear plastic eggshell hatching a tiny human being. Elizabeth ignores our patient for now, leaning on the incubator frame and making small talk, like we're chatting across the hood of her car.

"Eclipse?" I ask blankly, grabbing a pair of sterile gloves for the upcoming procedure.

"*You haven't* heard." Her voice holds that familiar note of smug confidence, the same tone she has used to lecture me on ventilator flow rates, newborn caloric requirements, and oxygen toxicity.

It's a tone I've grown quite used to lately. I had the incredible bad luck to start my first month of internship in the "nick-you," the Neonatal Intensive Care Unit. Worse yet, I drew Dr. Elizabeth "Hewlett" Packard as the unit chief resident, a walking, talking computer, with about the same amount of personality and charm. It's been an exercise in humiliation.

"It's just an annular one," Elizabeth clarifies, and I'm still not sure if she's talking about our patient or the eclipse. I glance down at Baby Johnson for a clue, but his wide blue eyes are fixed on Elizabeth, lips pulled taut in a gumless grimace of apprehension. He's been here long enough to know what's coming.

"I'll handle this one, alone," she mutters to me as I pull the gloves on. She pops open a fresh iv kit and opens the round incubator portals on her side. "B.J.'s pretty easy. Next time, I'll let you try him."

I know I should feel grateful, but I'm hoping there won't *be* a next time, that B.J. will be discharged before he needs another iv.

Reaching inside, Elizabeth pats her victim's chest absently, a token effort at soothing that B.J. isn't buying. He wriggles and kicks beneath her hand, but Elizabeth doesn't notice.

"Annular eclipses are ring-shaped, not quite complete." She peers at the butterfly needle and nods, a high priestess preparing her sacrifice. With deft precision, she probes Baby Johnson's head with the needle, puncturing a scalp vein made all the more prominent by the victim's struggles. "Should be quite a sight, though."

She reaches for the surgical tape, but B.J. suddenly twists like a gaffed salmon. The catheter slips from the vein, painting a trail of bright red blood across the sterile white sheet. A tiny hand clutches one of the wires, pulling it free and setting the heart monitor into a fit of frantic chirping. Inside the plastic bubble, B.J.'s mouth pitches wide to scream, but all we hear is a pitiful bleat, like a muzzled lamb.

Elizabeth shoots me a look of exasperation. The wave of satisfaction I feel at her blunder is swallowed by an undertow of guilt. Poor B.J.'s pinched purple face is screwed into a mask of fear and anger and pain.

I open another door and reach in to pat his chest, try to calm him while Elizabeth readies another kit. Poor little spud. Beneath my hands, B.J.'s ribs feel like the wires of a birdcage, his heart like fluttering wings struggling to break free. His tiny fingers spring shut on my thumb with surprising strength. Two weeks old, B.J. only weighs about four pounds, pencil-thin arms and legs jabbed into a shriveled pumpkin body. Still, B.J. outweighs most of the others here at the NICU.

To my surprise, he hiccups and calms down, squinting through the plastic wall and fixing on my face just as Elizabeth stabs another vein. He howls and squirms again, but we're ready for him this time. I clamp his arms and legs to the little plastic mattress while Elizabeth does the deed, thrusting with the steel catheter, slipping the plastic tube inside the vein, and taping the line down tight, all in one smooth motion.

I snap the monitor lead back onto his flailing chest. Between screams, his eyes open and he finds my face again. I pull a pair of sock-like gloves over his tiny hands and wipe the blood from his face, trying to ignore the accusation in his eyes.

"It's okay, B.J." I pat his tummy gently, forcing a plastic smile through the plastic window. "It's okay, little pal."

"He can't hear you," Elizabeth points out, ever the scientist. "The glass is too thick."

Still, B.J. quiets down, closes his eyes. He tires easily, more than you'd expect from a four-pounder born just six weeks early. But he has a nasty heart problem, too: the blood vessels leading out from his heart are all crossed up, so that oxygenated blood heads back to his lungs again, rather than out to the body.

"Everything's gonna be all right," I murmur, half to myself.

"Maybe, maybe not," Elizabeth shrugs, snapping her bloody gloves into the trash. "Depends on how the surgery goes. I'm scrubbing in—should be a fascinating case."

B.J.'s moment of truth would come tomorrow morning. Without the surgery, he probably wouldn't last more than another month or two. But if he survives, he could end up leading a pretty normal life, just like any other kid.

Our next patient isn't going to live a normal life, or any kind of life at all, most likely. Baby Sullivan's bubble is tucked away in an alcove near the Unit's only window, the best seat in the house. The window spot is available on a first-come, first-served basis. Newcomers start near the door, and we all hope they're discharged before they make it to the window. Only the long-term cases ever make it to the window spot, the tiniest premies with the flawed lungs and ailing hearts, spidery bodies and brains often maimed beyond hope of recovery.

Only a very few have ever made it home from the window seat. Up here on the twelfth floor, one step closer to the window is generally one step closer to heaven.

As usual, Frank Sullivan is parked in the big oak rocking chair beside his son's incubator. Despite his weeks of vigil in the Unit, he still looks utterly out of place here. A huge redheaded sequoia of a man, Frank is the kind of guy you expect to see doing home improvement shows or tossing cabers on public television. His red flannel shirt and blue jeans poke out from the sterile yellow smock that's always three sizes too small. A woolly red beard covers most of his face, but the rest of his head is as perfectly bald as his son's. Except, of course, Frank's doesn't have an IV.

He's snoozing in the rocker, beard pillowed on his chest, but his head pops up as we approach. He beams.

"I've been waiting for you to come by. Got something to tell you." He lays a massive paw on his son's incubator; Baby Sullivan's entire body could fit in the palm of his father's hand. "Bobby opened his eyes a little this morning. Smiled at me, I think."

"Did he really?" Elizabeth's dark eyes are fixed on the chart. "That's encouraging."

Her voice sounds mechanical, and not very convincing. But I can't blame her. Sir Laurence Olivier himself couldn't have faked optimism over the case. Bobby was born fifteen weeks early and barely weighed two pounds. As Elizabeth once put it, about the same as a Triple Burger at Wendy's, or one of those little roasting chickens you get at the grocery store.

He hasn't changed much in his first month of life. Every ounce gained has been a struggle, a race against time for Bobby's tiny body, lung maturity pitted against blindness from too much oxygen, liver function battling jaundice and brain damage, digestion of critically needed calories staving off colitis and infection.

But Bobby has been losing the race: the poor kid is only halfway around the track, and Death is grinning at the finish line.

"Finally got his room fixed up yesterday," Frank tells me with a wink. "We're doing it in Disney: Winnie-the-Pooh wallpaper, a Mickey Mouse lamp, Chip n' Dale curtains. Soon as Bobby gets home . . ."

"Did Doctor Randall talk to you about the EEG?" Elizabeth asks suddenly. She clips the chart back onto the rail and dons a fresh pair of gloves for the exam.

"No. Not yet!" Frank's beard swallows his smile. He rubs his forehead, suddenly looking tired. "Delores went home for a nap. We're going to talk to Doctor Randall after lunch today."

Delores Sullivan has spent most of her maternity leave in the rocking chair next to Bobby. Frank works the night shift at Lordstown, then drives out here in the morning so Delores can get some rest at home. One of them has been here, day and night, ever since Bobby first arrived.

A few of the other kids' parents come in once a week or even less, and I wonder why it has to be *this* baby, *these* parents.

Elizabeth checks the pulse oximeter on Bobby's finger. Its red laser light makes his whole finger glow like E.T.'s: "*Oouuchh.*" The rest of him looks pretty alien, too; it's hard to see the baby under there. We're treating his jaundice with ultraviolet light; it gives his near-translucent skin a surreal glow, and makes the teddy bears on his diaper shimmer in some weird purple color. The nurse put cotton balls on his eyes for the treatment; they sparkle a bright iridescent white. A narrow-gauge nasogastric tube thin as a fishing line forms an "S" curve along his cheek before disappearing into his nose. The endotracheal tube in his slack mouth lurches with each ventilation; his chest rises and falls in quick mechanical huffs and sighs. The rest of him is buried under a tangle of wires and leads and feeding tubes, monitor patches, and ID bracelets. It's a wonder any light can reach him under there.

Elizabeth goes through the motions of the exam while I get a suction kit ready for cleaning out the breathing tube. I drop the tubing down his throat to clear the secretions, brushing Bobby's leg with the side of my hand.

"There—see?" Frank peers over my shoulder, pointing a trembling finger. "See? He moved."

"It could have been a spinal reflex," Elizabeth starts to explain.

"No—I bumped his leg." Behind me, Frank doesn't seem convinced, so I do it again. "Like that. It was an accident."

"Well, he *did* move this morning." Frank slumps back into his chair again, broad shoulders drooping. "You folks know how the EEG came out?"

"No," we lie, and finish our exam. Frank doesn't say another word, and we slink away. I'm feeling guilty, and even Elizabeth is quiet for a while.

We spend the rest of the morning and half the afternoon making rounds with Dr. Randall, the neonatologist who's running the unit this month. He's about a hundred years old but still sharp as a tack, wizened and stooped and regaling us with stories from the pre-antibiotic era one moment, and quoting from this month's *New England Journal* the next. Easily the best teacher I've ever had, Dr. Randall is the idol of half the medical staff, and I'm ashamed to display my ignorance in front of him.

He goes easy on Elizabeth, since she's chief resident and knows all the answers anyway. As the only intern on the service this month, I get to field questions about oxygen flow rates, feeding tubes, gestational age, and about three dozen other things. By the time we're finished, my head is whirling with names and terms and equations, and I'm sure I've made a complete idiot of myself.

But Dr. Randall isn't.

"Not bad, young sir." In Dr. Randall's Unit, all the residents are young sirs and young misses. He beams and pats my arm. "Not bad at all. We'll make a neonatologist out of you yet."

Elizabeth smiles her approval. To celebrate, we head down to the cafeteria for a late lunch. It's after two o'clock, and the cafeteria is deserted—except for Delores Sullivan. She waves us over to her table, and we head across to set our trays down.

"Hi." Delores's mouth tightens in her best imitation of a smile. "You folks sure are eating late today."

Delores isn't eating at all. She's stirring some NutraSweet into a cup of black coffee. Over the past month, I've only seen her eat once: half a Twix bar that Frank forced on her. She's starting to look like one of the NICU kids—all angles and hollows and pale bluish skin.

We chat about the weather and Frank's job and the Cleveland Indians, wolfing our food in the minimum possible amount of time. Just as we're getting ready to leave, Delores drags out her real concern with a mixture of defiance and shame, like a kid pulling stolen candy from his pocket.

"Doctor Randall talked to us this afternoon."

Elizabeth surprises me, setting her tray down and sitting back patiently. She studies Delores with a sympathetic gaze. "What did he say?"

"Says Bobby's been in a coma." She frowns into her coffee, takes a little sip. "I guess we knew—you been telling us that all along. But we didn't want to believe it, especially Frank. You know how he is."

"I know."

She reaches out and pats Delores's hand, surprising me again. This is a side of Elizabeth I've never seen before. She has always seemed so competent, cold and clinical—one of those doctors who views illness and death as personal affronts, insults to their professional abilities.

"He said something about the eyes that I didn't understand," Delores continues. "I thought Bobby's problem was with his lungs."

"Bobby has a lot of problems—all premature babies do," Elizabeth explains patiently. In a quiet voice, she gently unravels the complex knot of diagnosis and treatment, telling Bobby's mother how too much oxygen can damage his eyes, but too little can damage his brain. How we try to walk the fine line between them, but sometimes end up having to choose one or the other, especially in babies as small as Bobby.

"So Bobby might have trouble seeing, when he comes home?"

When he comes home. I grimace, wondering when Delores and Frank will finally hear what we're saying.

"Did Doctor Randall talk to you about the EEG they did yesterday?" Elizabeth asks.

"Yes." Her brown eyes sink even deeper as she squints into her coffee. "He said it was just like the first one—almost flatline. Sounds like you folks have given up on Bobby."

She glares defiantly over the styrofoam rim.

"It's not a matter of 'giving up,' Delores," I protest. I hear the defensiveness in my voice; but I don't care. I've been on call four nights in the past week, thirty-six-hour days stuck in that beeping buzzing windowless prison, making rounds, answering alarms, shuffling through a haze of mind-numbing fatigue and doing the best I can to care for twenty-three pitifully small and helpless humans, and she talks about *caring.* God! "It's a matter of facing the facts. Bobby . . ."

I feel Elizabeth's hand on my arm, a gentle urgent pressure.

"Did Doctor Randall explain what that means?" she asks.

"Almost no brain activity." Delores shakes her head urgently. "But what if Bobby was asleep? My sister's baby sleeps sixteen hours a day. I bet Bobby sleeps a lot too. People can sleep in comas, can't they?"

"Maybe they can." Elizabeth shrugs. "But the brain is very active, even during sleep—maybe more so, for some people. Folks show lots of brain activity during dreams, and even during dreamless sleep." She spreads her hands helplessly. "Even during a coma, the brain still shows some kind of activity."

"Bobby's brain has activity, right?" Delores asks hopefully. She's leaning over the table, studying our faces earnestly, looking for some kind of loophole in Elizabeth's relentless logic. "Doctor Randall said *almost* flatline."

"Yes and no." Slowly, gently, Elizabeth explains how the EEG only picked up activity in the brainstem, the primitive part of the brain that controls vital functions like breathing, digestion, and heartbeat. The rest of Bobby's brain— the part that handles sensation, movement, and thought—is gone.

"Is that what they call 'brain dead'?" Delores is looking for a name, a term, something she's heard before. Something to make sense of it all.

"Just about." She nods slowly. "Even if we could fix the rest of his body, get him off of life support, he'd have profound brain damage."

"He'd be a vegetable." The mother's voice is harsh, flat.

"Yes." Elizabeth swallows heavily. "I'm sorry."

We all look out the window at the courtyard below. Some kids from the psych ward are playing on the swings, the monkey bars, the teeter-totters. I realize I haven't been outside since I drove in yesterday morning. The sun wasn't even up then.

"We been trying real hard, me and Frank," Delores tells the window. "Couldn't get pregnant for the longest time, then I lost three in a row. Got them lumps on my womb."

"Fibroids," Elizabeth says.

"Yeah. Doctor says we shouldn't try anymore. Says I'm bleeding too much. Wants to operate, take everything out. He says the bleeding would stop, and my cycles wouldn't hurt so much. But I don't *care* about that." She reaches into her purse, dabs at her eyes with a Kleenex. "I haven't decided yet."

"It's a tough choice," Elizabeth admits.

"That's just what Doctor Randall said. About Bobby." Abruptly, she turns to face us again, eyes swollen and puffy, cheeks stained with tears. "Wants us to decide what to do. *Us*—me and Frank." She laughs hollowly. "Talked about it like we was picking curtains, or deciding what kind of minivan to get."

"I can't imagine what you're going through." Elizabeth's voice cracks, and she stares up at the ceiling, blinking and rubbing her eyes. "If there's any way I can help—"

"We asked Doctor Randall to decide *for* us, to tell us what to do. He said he couldn't. Sweet Jesus—how can he expect us to . . ." Her voice drops to a whisper, almost drowned out by the whine of the fluorescent lights overhead, the clatter of the ice machine. "Frank wants you to keep him alive as long as you can. His poor heart was like to break when Doctor Randall talked about quitting." She takes a deep breath. "But I'm afraid Bobby's suffering. Trying to break free, somehow."

Elizabeth nods slowly.

Delores stares out at the trees and grass below, the children playing together. "I keep having this dream about taking Bobby out of here. Outside. I'm holding him, and we're dancing in the sunshine."

Elizabeth doesn't say anything for a minute or two. Then she looks up and meets Delores's gaze. "It sounds like you know what you want to do."

"Yeah." Delores Sullivan knuckles her eyes and shrugs helplessly. "But I don't know how we could ever do it."

Four days later, we're fiddling with Baby Doe's vent settings, in the incubator next to Bobby's. Little Jane almost made it to the window, but it looks like she's turning the corner. We've been slowly backing down on the ventilator, as she has finally started breathing on her own.

"Today we go to full assist/control ventilation," Elizabeth tells me. "You know all about assist/control, right?"

We've got an audience: Delores Sullivan is sitting in the oak rocker, following our discussion. I wonder if she is envious, if she knows that Baby Doe was found on the steps of St. Joe's Church over in Austintown. She must have noticed that nobody has ever come to visit the little premie in the unit beside her son.

And she must have wondered, as I had, why Jane Doe had turned the corner, and not Bobby Sullivan. Who makes these decisions, I wonder, then drag my mind back to ventilator settings. "With assist/control, the ventilator senses the baby trying to breathe, and delivers a breath for her."

"What's the point?" Elizabeth challenges. She's back to her usual self, tough as nails. Her talk with Delores the other day might never have happened. "Why not just use controlled ventilation?"

"Assist/control cuts down on the amount of work the baby has to do, but allows her to start controlling her own breathing."

"Good." She finally stops the inquisition and shows me how to drop the backup rate down to zero; now the machine won't deliver any breaths unless Baby Doe makes an effort first. Elizabeth checks the pulse oximeter on the baby's finger, then turns up the alarms for the oxygen level and pulse rate. "We want to be able to hear these. We'll stick around for a while, keep an eye on her and make sure everything's okay."

We move over to Bobby's incubator, and Elizabeth shows me the vent settings and controls. "Bobby's on assist/control too, see? Only difference is, his backup rate is set to sixty breaths per minute. Because he's not making any efforts to breathe, the machine is delivering all the breaths on its own."

She points to the dial that controls the backup rate. "Now, if we were going to wean Bobby, we'd slowly back this down to zero. Of course, the blood oxygen would drop and trigger the alarm, so we'd all come running."

She's stating the obvious now, but I just nod my head and feign interest.

"Ever wonder what your oxygen saturation is?" she asks me.

I grin. "After being on call last night, I'd guess it's about thirty percent."

Elizabeth opens a cupboard, finds one of the pulse oximeters, unplugs

Bobby's monitor cable, and replaces it with the new one. She presses it to my finger and we all glance up at the monitor: "Not even close—you're ninety-nine percent. Normal."

"I don't feel normal."

Delores smiles at us, one of her first smiles in weeks.

Elizabeth switches the lead back, leaving the extra oximeter on the counter near Bobby's incubator.

"Frank's not coming today?" she asks Delores.

"No. He's working a double shift."

"Then he'll miss the eclipse," Elizabeth notes. She cocks her head at Delores. "Have you heard about it?"

"No."

"It's all Elizabeth's talked about this week," I grumble. "She should have gone into astronomy."

"Nonsense," Delores says. "She's a fine doctor, one of the best I've ever met."

I'm surprised at the intensity of her remark, especially considering the object of her praise. Elizabeth?

"The eclipse starts at two-fifteen," she stammers. Astonishingly, the infamous Dr. Hewlett-Packard, as cold and emotionless as a computer hard drive, is actually blushing at the compliment. "You won't be able to see it from this window, though. Sun's on the other side of the building. We'll probably all be sneaking up to the balcony to take a look. This place'll be half deserted."

"What's the big deal?" I ask later as Elizabeth drags me up the last flight of stairs. "I've got eight more notes to write, and a pile of chartwork waiting for me down in medical records. I don't have time to sit around staring at the sky."

"How many eclipses have you seen?" she asks me.

I shrug.

"None, huh?"

"It probably slipped my mind."

"The next annular eclipse isn't for another nineteen years," Elizabeth points out. "You could be dead by then."

"Thanks for the cheery thought." But I grin, surprised at yet another new dimension of my chief resident's personality. She leads me to the door, positively giggling with anticipation of the event, and I realize that I'm only just beginning to know Elizabeth Packard, discovering that the brutally competent doctor in the NICU isn't she, or is only just a small part of the whole.

She swings open the door to the balcony, and it's like stepping into a party. Half the hospital staff must be up there. I see several other residents, a handful of nurses from the NICU, and even Doctor Randall. Elizabeth hands me a pair of special green-filtered glasses, and I glance up at the sun. Most of it is already shadowed by the lunar disc, but it's not quite centered yet. Through the glasses, the sun looks like a very bright crescent moon.

"Cool."

"See?" Elizabeth asks, patting my shoulder. We watch together as the eclipse approaches its maximum depth; then she takes her glasses off and gestures. "Check it out."

I pocket my glasses and look around, gasping at the stillness, the strangeness of the world. The downtown scene looks grayish-yellow and overcast, though the sky is completely free of clouds. The usually raucous mourning doves and pigeons have gone silent, the crowd on the balcony is hushed, and even the traffic below seems to slow and halt. Time itself seems to grind to a stop, and a sudden chill blows through the air.

I look around the balcony at the other doctors and nurses, hospital administrators, and cafeteria staffers, all equally amazed at the spectacle. I spot Dr. Randall again, standing on the other side of the roof beside a pair of nurses, doubtless regaling them with stories of the past dozen eclipses.

And then I remember. "Damn!"

"What?" Elizabeth frowns, concerned.

"Doctor Randall asked me to turn down Baby Johnson's IV this morning." I press the sunglasses into Elizabeth's hand. "I'd better do it before he gets back down there."

She tries to stop me, but I spring away and hurdle through the door. Behind me, the eclipse is reaching its peak, but I can't worry about it. Doctor Randall would chew me out for an hour if he knew I forgot about the IV.

I burst through the doors of the NICU and charge over to B.J.'s incubator, only to find that Elizabeth already dropped the flow rate. Most of the staff is upstairs; only one nurse is there, feeding one of the bigger babies in the windowed-off "growing" portion of the unit.

She gives me a funny look, so I dart into the intensive section like I have something important to do, just in time to see Delores Sullivan hunched over Bobby's incubator, one hand clasping his tiny tiny hand, the other holding the extra pulse oximeter against her finger. She turns and looks at me furtively, like a prisoner caught jumping the fence, and her eyes are full of tears.

In that moment, everything suddenly makes a crazy sort of sense. Elizabeth's lecture on the ventilator settings, though she knew I understood them already. Her little game with the pulse oximeters, even telling Delores about the eclipse.

I think for what seems like an hour but is only a few seconds, a crystallization of my short medical career. My very first patient, the charming and elderly Victoria Vandenberg, who died of incurable bone cancer one week after attending my graduation. The teenage hemophiliac with AIDS who kept asking me "why," as though they taught us those answers in medical school. Lectures on drugs and disease that ignored the fact that medicine often fails, that sometimes death is less of an enemy than doctors.

And finally, I come to the decision that every physician must face sooner or later, regardless of the path they ultimately choose.

I look away, pick an incubator at random, glancing down at the baby's chart and pretending Delores Sullivan isn't even there. Wondering again why it had to be *that* baby and *those* parents. Wondering why it had to happen at all.

An hour later, I'm back on the roof alone. The heart monitor finally went off, of course. I rushed over and pretended not to notice Delores reconnecting Bobby's pulse oximeter, while the nurse called a Code Blue that cleared the balcony like a cat among a flock of pigeons. Not that it mattered; Delores had gotten Frank to sign a "Do Not Resuscitate" order, so we all just stood around the bedside to watch Bobby fade away, the bright little squiggles on his heart monitor flattening out until he was finally and certainly gone.

Standing at the far edge of the balcony, I see the door open and a trio emerge into the light, Dr. Randall and Delores and Frank, who had rushed in from Lordstown to say goodbye. Frank is huddled protectively over his wife, both still dressed in their sterile yellow smocks, looking shaken but resolute. Delores is holding an impossibly small bundle of blankets; as she moves closer to the rail, I see her smiling through tears at the growing brightness of the day.

The last blurry overcast is finally disappearing. I put on the shades and watch as the moon finally delivers up the sun, disappearing in the brightness of its offspring. I hear footsteps behind me, feel a hand on my shoulder.

"It's funny," I tell Elizabeth. "Everything seems brighter, somehow. Clearer, and sharper."

"I know."

We stand there together, watching the city below us brighten and expand like an opening flower.

Dr. A. Makes Rounds

ABIGAIL DELL ZUGER

THE MONTH BEGAN like any other—after so many years on the attending staff of the Institute, Martin's habits on the first day of his ward months were fixed. He left his office in the research wing promptly at 9:50 A.M. He stepped off the elevator onto the ward promptly at ten. He glanced down each of the long corridors extending from the elevator, then entered the doctor's room immediately to his right, preparing a smile for his new house staff team.

But on the first day of that particular month—and Martin remembers this clearly, even long after he has difficulty recalling whether Leora's eyes were black or brown—on that morning the little room they called the doctors' station was empty.

Martin walked through the open door promptly at 10:00 A.M. and found himself alone. His face fell. What an appalling mess. The state of the room was all the more repugnant in the face of his own gleaming freshness, stiff, white cotton coat buttoned to wrist and knee, his name in cursive red stitching on the breast. He had developed a pleasant ritual for the day before his two ward months a year, heading down to the hospital laundry for a crisp, newly starched white coat, sorting through the papers that had accumulated in the pockets of the old coat—keeping some, throwing out others—cleaning the head of his stethoscope with an alcohol wipe and coiling it into a welcoming pocket.

As the month progressed the new coat would become limp and dingy, its pockets distended with index cards, xeroxed articles, odd tongue depressors and cotton swabs. On the last day of the month he would take the coat off, and, holding it by the neck like a creature newly dead, hang it gingerly on the back of his office door. There it would remain undisturbed until the afternoon before his next month on service, when he would take the used coat down to the laundry, bring another stiff thick pure cotton coat up in its place, and configure it anew.

Martin looked around the empty doctors' station. It smelled repellently of ripe banana. He leafed through the debris on the nearest laminate counter, a jumble of lab slips, shrink-wrapped syringes, half-completed X-ray requisitions, and a tube of rusty-brown blood. A wad of cellophane-encased napkin and coffee stirrer packages from the deli crunched under his foot. On the windowsill lay half a doughnut and an open plastic cup of something that looked very much like urine. A large hand-written sign taped to the bottom of the X-ray view box reminded residents to complete their discharge summaries within six hours of patients' departures.

The view box itself was switched on, a glowing rectangle of hot white plastic on the wall. Martin switched it off. He looked around again expectantly for a note with his name on it, possibly propped against the telephone, possibly scotch-taped to the doorframe. There was no note.

At 10:05 Martin fished into the left-hand pocket of his coat, extracted a wad of clean latex gloves, peeled off two, put them on. He picked up the plastic cup with one hand and with the other the tube of old blood. He carried them both outside to the small sink near the nurses' medication closet, dumped the urine down the sink, then tossed the tube and the empty cup into the "infectious body wastes" container. He removed the gloves, tossed them into the regular garbage, and lavishly washed his hands.

It was 10:08.

He approached the only human being in sight, a nurse rapidly typing into a computer at the nurse's station.

"Excuse me," Martin said to her bent head. "I am Dr. Arrowsmith. I am attending on the ward this month." He paused.

She continued to type.

"Are there any messages for me?"

The nurse flickered him a look up and down. "Not that I know of," she said, turning back to her screen.

Martin hovered uncertainly behind her. He was never kept waiting on the first of the month, preceded by his reputation as he inevitably was. Long before they met him the residents would already have heard about him and his idiosyncrasies—the insistence on white coats, the ban on blue jeans, the antique habits of treatment. At some point in the last few decades he had become a fixture, cemented in the relics of a distant time. In fact, he was still perfectly vigorous.

He tried again. "Excuse me."

The nurse swiveled her seat a few degrees in his direction, eyes fixed on her computer.

"Have you seen the house staff?"

A shake of the glossy head.

"Is any of the patients particularly ill?"

A shrug.

"Have there been any emergencies?"

Another shake of the head, magenta-tipped fingernails tapping efficiently over the keyboard.

Martin went back into the doctors' station, half-closed the door behind him, drew out a chair, extricated a tissue from a new packet in his pocket, wiped a small sticky globule of something or other off the seat of the chair, sat down, and waited.

When the door crashed open at 10:26, he didn't move. For a split second the grinning fellow moving through the doorway kept talking, bellowing some pleasantry to the person behind him. Then he saw Martin and fell silent, and like an indrawn breath the silence flashed back down the line.

The four of them sidled in, disgraced. The last one, a large boy dressed in a short, tight jacket rivaling Martin's in its dazzling whiteness, was chewing an enormous mouthful of something.

A murmur of "sorry" filled the room. The chewing one could only gurgle and swallow. Martin heard him distinctly. Although their faces were only vaguely familiar to him, he could still sort them out immediately. The chewer at the end of the line was clearly a medical student, given away by the brilliance of his linen. The short stocky fellow who was first through the door, shirttails poking out of his pants and a stethoscope draped around his neck, was one of the interns. The dilapidated middle-aged woman behind him with a large chain of wooden spheres dangling from her neck was the other intern; Martin distinctly remembered her face from the photo passed around the Residency Admissions Committee Meeting last fall. She was an ex-nun, apparently, with a great deal of interest in combining the healing of the body with that of the spirit.

And the other female in the room was the third year supervising resident; Martin had seen her around the hospital but had had no dealings with her. She had an odd first name, he remembered, which in any case he would not be using. He made a point of maintaining formal address with the residents.

"I'm Dr. Tozer," the resident said now, extending a hand in his direction. "We're sorry we're late."

Martin shook the hand and released it. "Where were you, Doctor?" Sitting in the empty room he had become increasingly insecure and uneasy, actually on the verge of calling his office to make sure he was in the right place. Now he was coldly furious.

"We all had to go to Morning Report. The new rule, that everyone goes?" She shrugged in apology. "It ran late."

Martin now remembered this rule, the subject of some eloquent debate at the last Department of Medicine meeting. He had actually delivered most of the debate himself, with an impassioned and completely unsuccessful plea in favor of leaving Morning Report as it had always been—an event for senior residents only, a rite of passage. He had recreated his own acute consciousness of the privilege of sitting knee to knee with Liebland at the General, actually sitting down to discuss a case, rather than presenting to the professor while standing stiffly at the bedside. And sipping coffee at the same time—it had been quite intoxicating. Worth waiting for.

But now, of course, everybody sat from the very beginning, medical students, interns, they all sat and chomped and slurped and listened to some predigested pap about health maintenance, resource allocation, what have you. As if demolishing a piece of pastry while someone lectured you about pneumonia was half as instructive as sitting in the room of your own patient with pneumonia, listening to the chest, feeling the racing pulse, watching the ribs retract with every breath.

The team settled into chairs around the room, chastened and expectant. The male intern jiggled a leg and ruffled through a sheaf of pink papers on his clipboard. The medical student, last mouthful swallowed, carefully extricated an index card from his jacket and poised a pen over it. The nun stared into space, her stethoscope held firmly coiled in her lap with both hands. The resident Tozer swept most of the debris on the counters into the overflowing garbage can, which she then moved outside the doorway of the room, noticeably diminishing the odor of banana. She came back in, closed the door behind her, and sat down. All were silent. Martin cleared his throat and began.

He was Dr. Arrowsmith.

They nodded.

And they were . . . ?

"Dr. Prasad, intern."

"Dr. Sullivan, intern."

"Um, Michael Lippman, I'm a medical student."

"Leora Tozer." (Lee-ora, not Lola or Laura. Bizarre name.)

He would be rounding with them every morning for the month. He preferred to hear new cases first, and then to discuss follow-ups. Here were his office numbers and here was his home phone. He did not carry a beeper. They were to feel free to call him whenever they had a question. They were to remember that he was legally responsible not only for everything they did, but also for everything they thought. Weekday rounds would begin promptly at ten. Saturday rounds would begin at eight, Sunday at nine.

In the future, when Morning Report ran over time, they were to leave Morning Report early. They were to refer anyone who complained straight to Martin. Were there questions?

No questions.

Everyone on the team would wear a white coat. No one would wear blue jeans. No one would eat during rounds. No one would drink coffee. He expected them to present new cases at the patient's bedside, from memory. All follow-up cases would be discussed at the bedside. They would be seeing very little of this room for the rest of the month. Were there questions?

There were no questions, but he saw them sneaking each other the usual looks. Martin knew perfectly well that he was the only attending in the department, probably the hospital, and possibly the world, who still made rounds at the bedside. Not to mention the stipulations about food and drink. Everyone else simply tolerated the sips and drips and showers of crumbs during rounds. Some even let the detail men, those omnipresent leeches from the pharmaceutical houses, sponsor meals themselves. Martin would see them staggering into the hospital in the mornings, a gallon jug of orange juice in one hand, a damp paper bag redolent of fresh-baked bagel in the other, tugging behind them their black wheeled suitcases full of product flyers.

As far as Martin was concerned, breakfast was breakfast, rounds were rounds, and advertisement was advertisement. You couldn't teach the stately rhythms of academic medicine, the lessons of Osler and Penfield, to someone with a free bagel in one hand and a ballpoint pen blaring some drug's name in the other. Martin always took a certain grim pleasure at the beginning of each month watching the young contemplate their imminent starvation.

He paused and looked around the room. All were silent.

"Let's get started," he said. "How many patients do we have all together?"

"I have three, one is new," said the male intern. Martin glanced at the identification tag clipped to his belt. V. Prasad.

"I just have one," said the nun.

"That's it," the resident said.

Four patients on his team. Martin shook his head. Even last year, they were running a dozen or more; five years ago, it was two or three dozen. No wonder they had to manufacture educational conferences for these kids—no one let sick people rest in hospitals any more.

"Well," he said. "Slim pickings, eh?"

They smiled politely.

"All right," he said. "New one first. Then you'll tell me about the others. Where to?" He rose from his chair, started for the door. No one moved.

The intern Prasad cleared his throat. "We have the one new case this morning. She is a sixty-nine-year-old lady, Baxter Frances, patient of Dr. Kahn. But Dr. Arrowsmith, we can certainly go to bedside, 505A, but she will not be there, she is presently in PFT. What shall we do?"

In the old days, no patient was ever in pulmonary function testing. No patient was ever anywhere but right there in bed where they belonged, all of them lined up in long rows in the big drafty wards, waiting for the morning and evening processions of doctors and nurses to pronounce and minister, respectively. Now patients were booked for tests every waking moment. Get them in, run every possible test, and get them out, pronto. When you can't keep them home entirely, that is.

Martin had been known to rebel against this phenomenon by holding a morning's rounds alongside a series of empty rumpled beds, but frankly, even he was not quite sure of the point he was trying to make.

"We will stay here for the case," he conceded, sitting down again. "Then we'll go see the other patients."

"And we have Noon Lunch Conference," the medical student blurted out. "At noon," he added.

Martin gave him a look, then turned back to the intern. "Dr. Prasad. Please."

Twenty minutes later, Dr. Prasad had plowed through the story of Mrs. Baxter, a lady of many misfortunes, not the least of which, as far as Martin could make out, was her inexplicable loyalty to the ministrations of her private physician, Dr. Kahn. The intern finished reciting the results of a lengthy series of outpatient tests, all unnecessary as far as Martin was concerned, and then started on his assessment, reading directly from his pink sheets and sweating slightly.

"Problem number one: Fever. This lady has slight fever of less than 101. I believe this to be a fever of unknown origin. Because I do not know where it is coming from." He looked up, grinning. The others tittered. Martin registered a twinge of annoyance. "Fever of unknown origin" was no joke; it was a highly technical term for a very interesting problem, the subject of much of his own research in the fifties. Fever of unknown origin, he recited silently to himself: a fever lasting more than a month for which a competent medical investigation fails to find a cause. Not only had Mrs. Baxter had fever for a mere ten days, but her doctor was Dr. Kahn. So much for competent medical evaluation. Where to begin?

Martin opened his mouth, but Prasad, head bent back down over his pink sheets, had resumed.

"Although I believe the fever may come from urinary tract infection. UTI. These are common in women. We have the urine pending." He stopped, looked around briefly, deftly avoided meeting Martin's incredulous eye, looked back down at his pages, continued.

"Problem number two: Fatigue. It is possible that this lady is low in thyroid. Hypothyroid. This condition is common in women. It is common in elderly. It will cause fatigue. We have the thyroid blood tests pending. Problem number three: Breathing difficulty. There is no history of asthma. Still, it is possible that asthma has developed here. Although I did not hear a wheeze. But it might be there later. Dr. Kahn said do the pulmonary function testing, and then we will see. It is pending. Chest X-ray was done. It is downstairs. To me, it appeared normal. The exact official reading is pending."

He paused for breath, eyes on his papers, then finished up at top speed. "Problem number four: Anemia. This lady has a low red blood cell count, this may represent iron deficiency, which is common in women. And in elderly. We have drawn the tests; they are pending. Problem number five: Dental, very poor teeth and gums, extraordinarily so. Due to old age without a doubt. We have called the dentist; he is pending." Prasad shuffled his papers together and looked expectantly at Martin.

Martin was momentarily speechless. Every time he left the wards for a few months he forgot how bad it had all become. Although, to be fair, this fellow Prasad was a perfectly average specimen of his type, the new species of resident that the educators were churning out these days. Teach medicine over brunch and this was what you got: kids who could list problems and prescribe a pill for each, but couldn't think. It was a miracle the woman hadn't been given antibiotics for the urinary tract infection she didn't have, thyroid hormone for her nonexistent thyroid condition, asthma pump for her nonasthma, and sent out the door.

"Oh." Prasad slowly raised his hand just as Martin began to speak. "I forgot to say. Dr. Kahn has asked for her to be placed on treatment. I have given her iron, an asthma pump, and the new once-daily oral cephalosporin for complete antibiotic coverage. We think it may be the urine. This morning she is resting comfortably. Home tomorrow, perhaps!"

He nodded emphatically. A short silence ensued. The medical student had inched some sort of small machine out of his jacket pocket and began punching its keys, making annoying little cheeping noises with each punch. The nun was flipping through the small pocket formulary of drugs and drug doses that all the house staff carried. The resident looked out the window, inscrutable. A glitter in her profile caught Martin's attention. He looked more closely. A procession of silver hoops was marching up the cartilage of her left ear, and there was the definite suggestion of a small hole in the wing of her left nostril. And worst of all, she was silently, energetically chewing a wad of gum.

A global irritation seized Martin. Not only was he now doomed to cope with the problems of Mrs. Baxter all month—and his clinical instincts told him she was a sick and complicated case—not only was he condemned to be patient with this unfortunate intern and start his medical education all over again from the beginning, not only would he be fighting all month against the inroads of Morning Report on one end of his rounds and Noon Lunch Conference on the other, but now here was the resident on the team, his lieutenant, pierced like a cannibal and chomping.

"Do you have any thoughts, Dr. Tozer?" he asked coldly.

The resident turned back to face the room. Her glittering ear receded behind a wing of dark hair.

"Uh, I didn't see her yesterday, Dr. Arrowsmith," she said. "The resident downstairs covers me after five."

"You've heard the case," said Martin grimly. He suddenly wanted to confront all the month's bad news at once. "Summarize the case and tell us what you think."

The resident obediently glanced down at the index card in her hand, then looked back up straight at Martin.

"The patient is a sixty-nine-year-old woman who presents with fever for ten days, and lethargy, dyspnea, weakness for approximately two weeks. Her physical exam is notable for a low-grade fever of 100.2, rapid pulse, rapid respirations, normal blood pressure. She has extremely poor dentition, a soft systolic heart murmur, and clear lungs. I didn't hear anything about skin lesions or eye findings. Neurologic exam was normal. Her laboratories were notable for an abnormal urinalysis with red and white blood cells and no bacteria. She also has a normocytic anemia, a normal white cell, a slightly elevated platelet count, and normal electrolytes. Chest X-ray is reportedly normal."

"Good." Martin was impressed in spite of himself. A competent case summary in the classical style, with vital signs first, laboratories last, and the urinalysis right where it belonged. Perfect.

"So, go on," he said. "What do you think?"

"I guess the first thing I would think would be endocarditis," she said. "You know, from her teeth. Maybe she was at the dentist recently and forgot to mention it. Did anyone ask?"

Prasad looked guilty and shook his head.

"Endocarditis would account for all her problems," the resident said. "The fatigue and shortness of breath might be from anemia, or failure from a bad valve, or she might have pulmonary emboli that aren't visible on chest X-ray yet. For other diagnostic possibilities—an autoimmune or connective tissue disorder, such as polyarteritis nodosa; or she could have a malignancy of the kidney. Of course, TB is the most common cause of fever of unknown origin, but then, she doesn't really have a classical FUO, because for that you have to be documented febrile for four weeks, and she has only had a fever for ten days. And furthermore . . ."

After "furthermore," Martin briefly stopped listening. Furthermore! The pierced kid was saying all the right things. Martin couldn't have summarized the case better himself. The woman almost certainly had endocarditis, an infection in her heart, possibly carried there from her bad teeth. He started to listen again, just as the resident mentioned his own *Annals* paper from '65. Then she quoted from it. Accurately. Martin gaped at her. Finished, she looked back at him with a small smile. At the edge of her face the column of earrings glittered. She gave her gum a quiet chew. In spite of himself, Martin smiled back. Still smiling, he turned back to the unfortunate Prasad.

"That is an excellent synthesis of your case."

"Ah." Prasad nodded, clutching his pink sheets.

"Did Dr. Kahn think this patient might have endocarditis?"

"No . . . asthma, he says to me, hypothyroid . . ." Prasad trailed off.

"Doesn't it make more sense to give her one diagnosis instead of four?"

"Oh yes."

"Not to send this lady off for every test in the hospital before you think things through?"

"Yes indeed."

"Not to load her up with medicines first?"

"Oh yes."

"What do you think about ordering PFTs in a patient who may have endocarditis?"

Prasad paused for a moment. "Not good?"

Martin made a little beckoning movement with his hand, waits for more.

"Possibly, bad."

"A person with a large infection right in the middle of the heart, with infectious debris hanging off her heart valves, is sent to inhale and exhale as hard as she possibly can for an hour . . ."

"This is very bad, I think." Prasad stretched an arm towards the telephone lying on the counter.

"Oh, too late, too late," Martin said. "Did Dr. Kahn by any remote chance remind you to draw blood cultures before you put this lady on antibiotics?"

Without blood cultured for bacteria, a diagnosis of endocarditis would be impossible to confirm. Now that the woman had been dosed with one of those accursed broad-spectrum cephalosporin antibiotics, the chance of obtaining positive blood cultures was nil: the cultures would be sterilized by the antibiotic even if the heart infection was there.

"Oh yes." Prasad nodded emphatically.

"How many?"

"Four bottles," said Prasad. "I myself drew."

"What are our chances of making a diagnosis with only four bottles?" Martin looked around the room. Silence. "Dr. Tozer?"

"About eighty percent," she said with complete accuracy.

"If we had gotten six bottles?"

"About eighty-seven percent."

Martin stared at her. Right on target again.

"Dr. Arrowsmith?" It was the nun. "I don't understand why you think she has an infection. There aren't any bacteria in the urine. Doesn't that mean infection is unlikely?"

Martin cleared his throat to explain the urinary abnormalities in endocarditis. But the resident beat him to it, delivering a short but utterly complete discussion of immune complex glomerulonephritis. All Martin could do was nod from time to time. The nun took copious notes. Prasad, buoyant as a beachball, bounced back into the discussion.

"My patient is very depressed," he said sadly, looking around the room, "Very low indeed. I feel this must contribute to her condition." It proved that Mrs. Baxter lived alone in a fifth floor walkup apartment, ignored by her only son. The nun sighed and shook her head. The medical student suddenly looked up from his cheeping machine to announce that he had entered all the patient's signs and symptoms into the Mayo Clinic's new diagnosis program, and it had come up with a diagnosis of endocarditis. He caught Martin's eye and stuffed the machine back into his pocket, reddening.

The resident looked at her watch. Martin could feel the specter of Noon Conference breathing heavily down his neck. Somehow, though, he was no longer oppressed by the sum total of the month's aggravations. He felt cheerful and in control. He got to his feet and suggested that they all go meet Mrs. Baxter. They straggled out of the room and the resident steered them down the left-hand corridor with Martin close at her heels. The others lagged further and further behind. Turning to hurry them along Martin found them stopped ten yards behind, heads bent over the medical student's cheeping box.

Up ahead the resident was standing by a gurney parked along the corridor wall just short of the last doorway. On it, a tiny elderly black woman lay swaddled in a sheet, arms folded across her chest like a medieval saint's.

"Mrs. Baxter?" Martin said.

A scowl and a tiny nod. She was indeed Mrs. Baxter, back from the pulmonary function lab.

"Mrs. Baxter. I am Dr. Arrowsmith." Martin smiled and took one of her waxy hands in his own. "I am working with your young doctors here on the ward. How are you feeling this morning?"

Mrs. Baxter looked at him briefly, then looked away. The resident's beeper suddenly went off with a shriek. All three of them jumped, and Mrs. Baxter, face now turned firmly to the wall, began to cry.

She was not feeling well at all. She had been unable to blow into the machines in that icy cold room. She did not understand why she seemed to be meeting doctor after doctor, and yet not one of them was Dr. Kahn, her doctor. She had to go to the bathroom.

Martin made soothing noises, taking in with an expert eye her gray-tinged skin and lips, her rapid breathing. He folded the sheet back and placed his stethoscope briefly over her bony chest, hearing the whoosh of the heart murmur even through her calico hospital gown. He looked carefully at the fingertips of her right hand, still encased in his own, then looked wildly around for his team of doctors.

But Martin and Mrs. Baxter were suddenly alone together in the corridor. The cheeping threesome was still in a huddle way down the corridor. The resident was talking into a wall telephone ten feet off.

He had no one to show his discovery to. Even Mrs. Baxter had closed her eyes and retreated far away, leaving only her hand behind.

Martin looked at the hand again. A small collection of raised red knots were scattered on her doughy fingerpads, no more than six or seven. They were easy to overlook, unless you were looking for them. They were the skin lesions of endocarditis, discovered by the great Osler himself.

"Pathognomonic," Martin murmured to himself, holding the hand in his.

He actually had forgotten that he was holding a hand that was attached to Mrs. Baxter, whose only son no longer visited her. He saw only a tangled hand-shaped web of veins and venules and capillaries, like a computer-generated model, but one gone wrong. Some of the hair-fine lines under the skin of her fingers were plugged with infection, swollen and distorted, their branches shriveling beyond the swellings like dead tendrils of ivy. Way upstream, Martin knew, a leaky heart valve was struggling, its edges eroded by infection, its surface unnaturally pocked and jagged like the surface of the moon, littered with small hard pebbles of bacteria and white cells. With each heartbeat a dust-cloud of particles rose from the valve and went speeding into the circulation, moving through the large blood vessels but catching in the smaller ones, damming the free flow of blood behind and killing the tissue up ahead, each logjam turning into a small abscess deep in the netherworld of the body—in the brain, the kidney, the lung, and the gnarled fingers held in Martin's own.

Fifty years ago a rash like Mrs. Baxter's was a death sentence. Martin remembered those days well. And now six weeks of antibiotics would probably take care of her problem. If she needed a new valve, why, she would get one, as simple as that. A span of medical history in the palm of a hand. Every resident in the hospital should hold this hand. He looked wildly around again, just as the resident materialized at his side.

Wordlessly, Martin held the hand out to her.

Her eyes widened. "Oh, look at that," she breathed. She reached out to touch a gentle finger to Mrs. Baxter's fingertips. "I never saw them before. Unbelievable. Just like the pictures." She ran gentle fingers slowly up and down over the bumps.

"That was the lab on the phone," she said after a moment. "She's growing a strep in her blood. All of them." All of Mrs. Baxter's blood cultures were growing a bacteria that looked like a streptococcus, the most common cause of endocarditis. She had endocarditis. The diagnosis was made.

They smiled at each other again.

The interns and medical student hurried up to Mrs. Baxter's gurney.

"I fear it is time for Noon Conference," Prasad said.

Martin looked at him. "Did you notice her fingers?" he asked. Mrs. Baxter suddenly opened her eyes. "Is that my new little doctor? Hello Doctor," she said weakly. Her fingers, still encased in Martin's grip, waggled weakly at Prasad.

Prasad beamed at her, and waggled his own fingers back. "Hello there, Frances." Then he looked closely at her fingers. "I did not notice. What a funny rash. Shall we call the Derm to check it out? I will call after conference. But if I do not get to conference right now, all the pizza will be gone."

The resident nudged Prasad. "Just help me get her in bed before you go," she said. "But conference!" said Prasad.

"Go to the conference," Martin interrupted wholeheartedly, surprising himself. "Everyone go to conference. Dr. Tozer and I will finish up together."

The interns and the student gratefully disappeared. Martin took one side of Mrs. Baxter's gurney and the resident took the other; together they wheeled Mrs. Baxter into her room.

A Parable

Richard Selzer

WELL, NOT A REAL parable with a beginning, middle, and end. This is only the middle, the part that is taking place here and now.

The scene is a room at the hospital. I am standing in the open doorway. It is early morning. A man is lying in the bed. He is emaciated, his skin covered with purple blotches where the blood has leaked into the tissues and congealed there. He is motionless, inert. Only his breathing gives evidence of life. It comes in short, rapid bursts interrupted by long stretches of apnea as though a creature sat astride him and rode him until he could not take a breath. Then it would start in again. It is called Cheyne-Stokes respiration. When they start that, you know it won't be long. There is suppuration around his eyes, blocking his vision. He makes no effort to clear the phlegm rattling in his throat, only coughs mechanically now and then.

A doctor comes into the room. I step aside to let him pass. He is wearing a blue scrub suit as is worn in the operating theater. He is elderly, with hair the color of pewter and blue eyes. His arms are thin and hairless and white. They end in hands that seem too large and heavy for the arms. They are red and shiny from years of scrubbing with stiff brushes. He takes a tissue, moistens it, and wipes the purulence from the sick man's eyes. Now I can see that his eyes are dark, the color of wet stones. They move to bring the doctor into focus. From the doorway of the room where I am standing, I see the lips of the doctor move, but I cannot at first hear what he is saying. He bends closer, placing his mouth almost to the man's ear, and raises his voice. Now I hear a soft humming. During the night the patient has slid down in the bed and has gotten knotted among the sheets. The doctor slides one hand beneath the patient's hips and the other beneath his shoulders and lifts him up, embracing him, enclosing him as if his arms were a cloak or a hiding place where the man, in his misery, might rest safe and secure.

The man in the bed now tries to speak, but his voice is broken, fissured, bleeding, and he cannot. All that emerges from his mouth are syllables in their larval state, mangled, and coagulated in a viscous unintelligible soup. From where I stand, I imagine that the sick body is hot, so hot that it gives forth warmth, like a stone that has lain out in the sun. A steam seems to rise from the bed. The old doctor holds his hands over the body of the man as if to warm them. The man makes another effort to speak. When the doctor turns his head to bend an ear to the lips of his patient, I can see the deep furrow that divides his brow, extending from the bridge of the nose almost to the hairline. It gives his face a pained expression. It is a line of pain. Had he been born with it? I wonder. No, I think he had not. Rather, it had appeared on the day that he treated his first patient. At first, it was merely a shadow on his forehead, then a slight indentation that, over the years, has deepened into this dark cleft that is the mark of all the suffering he has witnessed over a lifetime as a doctor. It resembles a wound that might have been made with an ax.

Now the doctor lowers his hands into the heat and the steam and places them on the naked abdomen. Gently, he presses, palpating, all the while speaking. "Am I hurting you?" he asks, or is it the wide-awake hands that ask the question? Those same hands that only that morning had made an incision, then slipped into another belly, exploring, then stopping at the moment of the recognition that Death had already slipped His hand inside that abdomen to knot its coils of intestine, stud its membranous surfaces. The man in the bed shakes his head. All at once (who would have thought he had the strength?), he raises one trembling hand and moves it toward the doctor's head. Could it be that the doctor bends forward a little so as to bring his cloven brow within reach? The sick man finds the furrow with his finger, touches, then strokes it from one end to the other, a look of wonder upon his face, as though he were just waking from a deep sleep. As he does so, a spicule of light appears to emanate from the doctor's forehead. It is a warm light that grows to engulf the two men and the bed. From this touching, the doctor does not withdraw, but smiles down at the patient with his sapphiric gaze.

The doctor covers the man's abdomen, and lifts the sheet to expose his feet. They are blue and, I think, cold despite the fever. The doctor takes one foot in his hand and begins to massage it gently, the way you rub the blood into a frozen part of the body. The man closes his eyes as if to concentrate the comfort he feels. His breathing slows and eases. Within minutes, he is asleep.

From the doorway, the two men and the bed appear luminous. They exist in a miraculous light. Miraculous? Why not? There are certain moments of harmony and revelation when miracles might be expected. They seem right and proper, like the luminous glow that has appeared to envelop the sick man and his doctor so that they themselves seem to be composed of light. On the contrary, if there had been no miraculous light about them, it would have been astonishing.

It is as if I were witnessing a feast. As if a table has been set with linen and plates and silverware. Candles have been lit. Ah, so that is the source of the light! There is bread in a small basket, and wine in the goblets. The two men are dining together, each the nourishment of the other.

The doctor covers the man's feet, turns and walks towards the doorway. Once again I stand back to let him pass. I see he is bent, his fingers knotted, arthritic. He does not move his arms but lets them hang at his side. His gait is shuffling, hesitant. What is it that he is whispering to himself?

It is the next morning. I am once again standing in the doorway of that room. The doctor, dressed in the same blue raiment that matches the color of his eyes, is making his rounds. He walks up to the bed where the man is lying perfectly still. His fingers reach for the man's wrist. He draws down the covers and observes the chest and the face, places his palm over the man's heart. Now he reaches up and closes the patient's eyes. With this small gesture, he sends the dead man on his way. As he leaves the room, it seems the furrow is not quite so deep and dark as on the day before.

Notes on Contributors

๛

Rafael Campo is a faculty member and practices general internal medicine at Harvard Medical School and Beth Israel Deaconess Medical Center. His latest collection of poems, titled *Diva*, was a finalist for the National Book Critics Circle Award, the Paterson Poetry Prize, and a Lambda Literary Award.

Robert Coles is a child psychiatrist and a faculty member at Harvard University. The author of more than fifty books, he won the Pulitzer Prize for his book series *Children of Crisis* and is the best-selling author of *The Spiritual Life of Children* and *The Call of Service.*

Jack Coulehan is the director of the Institute for Medicine in Contemporary Society and a professor of medicine and preventive medicine at the State University of New York at Stony Brook. He is the author of two collections of poetry, *The Knitted Glove* and *First Photographs of Heaven*, and co-editor of a collection of poems written by physicians, *Blood and Bone.*

Elissa Ely practices psychiatry at a state hospital in Massachusetts. She is a commentator for National Public Radio's *All Things Considered* and a contributing writer of the Editorials/Op-Ed section for the *Boston Globe.*

F. Gonzales-Crussi is a faculty member at Northwestern College of Medicine. He is the author of numerous books, including *Notes of an Anatomist, Three Forms of Sudden Death and Other Reflections on the Grandeur and Misery of the Body, On the Nature of Things Erotic, The Day of the Dead,* and *Other Mortal Reflections.*

David Hellerstein is a psychiatrist and clinical director of the New York State Psychiatric Institute at Columbia Presbyterian Medical Center. He is author of *Battles of Life and Death; Loving Touches;* and *A Family of Doctors,* which recounts five generations of physicians in his family. He has recently published an e-novel, *Stone Babies.*

David Hilfiker was a family practitioner in rural Minnesota and later was the medical director of Columbia Road Health Services in Washington, D.C. His *Not All of Us Are Saints* describes his work with homeless men dying of AIDS. *Healing the Wounds* was awarded first prize by the American Medical Writers Association.

PERRI KLASS is a pediatrician in Boston. Her novels include *Other Women's Children* and *Recombinations*. She recounts the trials and tribulations of medical school, internship, and residency in *A Not Entirely Benign Procedure* and *Baby Doctor*.

JOHN LANTOS is associate director of the MacLean Center for Clinical Medical Ethics and chief of general pediatrics at the University of Chicago, and has a clinical practice at the La Rabida Hospital, a specialty hospital for children with chronic disease. He is the author of *Do We Still Need Doctors?* and *A Tiny Baby in the Court of Law*.

SUSAN ONTHANK MATES is a retired physician and a former clinical associate professor of medicine at Brown University. She is the author of numerous short stories and essays. A collection of her short stories, titled *The Good Doctor*, won the John Simmons Fiction Award.

FITZHUGH MULLAN is a clinical professor of pediatrics and public health at the George Washington University, a member of the medical staff at the Upper Cardozo Community Health Center in Washington, D.C., and is a contributing editor of the journal *Health Affairs*. His books include *White Coat Clenched Fist: The Political Education of an American Physician*, and *Big Doctoring: Primary Care in America*.

WILLIAM J. POMIDOR is a graduate of the Northeastern Ohio Universities College of Medicine, where he is currently a faculty member. He is the author of several novels, including *Murder by Prescription*, *The Anatomy of Murder*, *Skeletons in the Closet*, *Ten Little Medicine Men*, and *Mind Over Murder*. He was nominated for an Edgar Award.

MAUREEN RAPPAPORT is a family physician in private practice in Montreal, the clinical supervisor of palliative home care at St. Mary's Hospital, and an assistant professor of family medicine at McGill University. Her prose and poetry have been published by the *Canadian Medical Association Journal* and the *Canadian Family Physician*.

L. J. SCHNEIDERMAN is a professor of community and family medicine at the University of California at San Diego. He is author of a novel titled *Sea Nymphs by the Hour* and has written numerous prize-winning short stories and plays.

RICHARD SELZER is a retired professor of surgery from the Yale Medical School. He is the author of several books, including *Mortal Lessons*, *Taking the World in for Repair*, and an autobiography—*Down from Troy*. He has won a National Magazine Award, an American Medical Writers Award, a Guggenheim, and a fellowship at Yaddo.

SAMUEL SHEM (STEPHEN BERGMAN) is a faculty member at Harvard Medical School. He is the author of several novels, including *The House of God* and *Mount Misery*, and a play about the formation of Alcoholics Anonymous, *Bill W. and Dr. Bob*.

JOHN STONE is a cardiologist and professor at Emory University School of Medicine. He has written four collections of poetry: *In All This Rain, Renaming the Streets, The Smell of Matches,* and *Where Water Begins.* His prose writing is collected in *In the Country of Hearts: Journeys in the Art of Medicine.*

ABIGAIL DELL ZUGER, a specialist in infectious diseases, is an associate clinical professor of medicine at the Albert Einstein College of Medicine in New York. She is the author of several articles about medicine and health care and a book titled *Strong Shadows: Scenes from an Inner City AIDS Clinic.*

Permissions

❧

Index

◆